FORWARD FROM THE MIND

Distant Healing, Bilocation, Medical Intuition & Prayer In a Quantum World

FORWARD FROM THE MIND

Distant Healing, Bilocation,
Medical Intuition & Prayer
In a Quantum World

Tiffany Snow

Spirit Journey Books
San Diego, California

FORWARD FROM THE MIND
Distant Healing, Bilocation, Medical Intuition & Prayer
In a Quantum World
Copyright © 2006 Tiffany Snow

Printed in the United States of America
First Edition

Unless otherwise identified, Scripture taken from the HOLY BIBLE, New International Version ®. Copyright © 1973, 1978, 1984 by International Bible Society. Used by permission of Zondervan Publishing House. All rights reserved.

Published by
Spirit Journey Books
P.O. Box 61
San Marcos, CA 92079

www.SpiritJourneyBooks.com

Toll-Free 1(800) 535-5474
The Divine Wellness Institute

For more information regarding
Miracle Healings please visit:

www.TiffanySnow.com

Edited by:
Billy Clark O.H.C.C.
Cover Design by:
Trish Wallace & Cat Stevenson

Library of Congress Catalog Number: 2006907662
International Standard Book Number
ISBN 978-0-9729623-6-0

1. Spirituality. 2. Alternative Medicine: Health, Mind & Body

DEDICATION

What a journey it has been,
And continues to be!
For you, my Holy One
Mean everything to me.

I feel like a tiny raindrop
Falling into the vast sea.
For I do not lose myself,
But become fully free.

And the ocean as well
I have come to intimately see
Is also Love's raindrop
Where "I" becomes "We."

TIFFANY SNOW carries the Holy Stigmata upon her body, and is an Evidence-based Miracle Healer, Award-winning Author, Medical Intuitive and Public Speaker. She has been called a Modern-Day Mystic, along the spiritual paths of Teresa of Avila or Padre Pio. Tiffany simply calls herself, "A Worker for The Big Guy." Her near-death experience by lightning-strike seven years ago blew "God out of the box," and experiencing the stigmata consistently since July of 2005 has led to empirical revelations beyond religion of habit. This includes clarity about quantum mechanics, methods of bilocation, remote viewing and distant healing. She shares that God is beyond religion, Love is beyond fear, and that miracles can be common place in every life, every day.

"Blessed Tiffany," as many lovingly call her, offers profound spiritual insight into how and why compassion and specific intention and prayer can become a place of Connection that bridges space and time, where heaven touches earth, and changes manifest before human eyes. This is a place where anything can happen, and often does – whether it is moving a pencil across the desk with the mind, miraculous healings or being witnessed on another side of the world through bi-location.

You won't find Blessed Tiffany in white billowy dresses, separating and elevating herself above others and belting out a religious agenda – instead, you will find her wearing green or blue nurse "scrubs," while working and moving among people of all faiths, beliefs and non-belief systems, as she helps and inspires through words and miraculous healings for all. Blessed Tiffany is able to help people make connection and see the potential each has to accomplish all the dreams and desires of their heart, as they develop a mind of tranquility and gratitude in the empowerment of Love.

Blessed Tiffany draws people to her like moths to a flame. They come to feel her warmth, be healed by her hands, and bask in the glow of her simple communion with God. All the while, she teaches and encourages – her words are peaceful and genuine. She gently reminds people that she is not special or in any way different from any of them, that none of us are greater or lesser than anyone else, that we are all in this together. She tells them, "I am a child of God...just like you! We are the same. We all have Gifts, we are all Loved!"

In New Mexico she was welcomed and accepted in a Pueblo Indian reservation to work side-by-side with their local medicine woman; in the hollows of Kentucky she was "adopted" by locals to heal their farms - all inclusive of people, horses, dogs and cats. In the Bible Belt of Tennessee, she was quietly brought into hospitals and churches to heal the sick and infirm. In Hawaii, she gave astonishing and validated information on

Hawaiian history and archeology, as she also did in Tennessee and New Mexico. She has helped on missing person and murder cases, and with the FBI on 9/11. She is also a medical intuitive and successfully heals with miracles by long-distance, as a preliminary research study and letters and emails from all parts of the world confirm. As Blessed Tiffany says: "God knows where everybody is, why place limits on Him?"

Blessed Tiffany was born in Vista, California. As an only child, she grew up living all over the country and traveling the back roads of the American Dream. She started writing, playing instruments and painting as a child, and would spend countless hours in nature where wild animals often joined her companionship and song. She later went on to care for and rehabilitate many wounded creatures which were rescued and brought to her by the US Forest Service and BLM.

Blessed Tiffany's desire to know "beyond" and understand "the bigger picture" started her on a spiritual quest from her earliest years; culminating in religious ordination before 20 yrs old. Through the years she raised four children nearly single-handedly through bouts of poverty, broken marriages, and trauma and abuse of all kinds. She persevered and went on to produce several instrumental and country albums, toured as a musician extensively, and found that her life of personal brokenness gave her insight of compassion for others and activated her prayer life. She came off the road shortly before the lightning strike which stimulated a brand new avenue of her life's awakening adventure.

The detailed information received during Blessed Tiffany's stigmata is really helping the world. And she is sharing it through books, healing prayer classes, workshops and speaking/healing events. She still songwrites, composes and paints - now of the dimensions and wonders she sees beyond, in a quest to manifest Father's love and compelling the invisible to the visible for the human eye, ear, and heart. She lives in Southern California with her husband, where they continue to witness miracles everyday in her healing prayer work at The Divine Wellness Institute in Escondido, California. 800.535.5474 www.TiffanySnow.com

CONTENTS

REVIEWS - FORWARD FROM THE MIND

"Tiffany Snow had a near-death experience that changed her life. She came out of it with amazing paranormal abilities. The present book, **Forward From the Mind,** not only details these abilities but gives the reader the knowledge and techniques to learn and use them for the betterment of humanity. These abilities include psychometry, remote viewing (especially for medical intuition), distant healing, both spiritual (with techniques such as Reiki, Therapeutic Touch and Quantum Healing) and prayer. We also learn about out-of-body experiences, stigmata and bilocation. Dr. Snow gives us the scientific and spiritual background for these paranormal abilities. An easy-to-understand discussion is given of quantum theory and its application to paranormal phenomena. I highly recommend this book for religious observers, people interested in the paranormal, individuals who require healing, skeptical scientists, and any other true skeptic. In other words, this book would prove beneficial for those who want to learn how to help others as well as themselves."

Donald R. Morse, DDS, PhD
Editor-in-Chief
The Journal of Religion and Psychical Research

"Tiffany Snow has produced a remarkable book unlike any other. Whereas most books on healing rely on selected testimonials for support, **Forward From the Mind – Distant Healing, Bilocation, Medical Intuition & Prayer in a Quantum World** includes a wealth of in-depth questionnaire data that not only establish the effectiveness of Snow's healing but also permit insights into how it works." *(Bruce is one of the first founding fathers of NDE research to gather empirical data using accepted scientific methods; past president of IANDS. He also reviewed our preliminary LD study.)*

Bruce Greyson, M.D.
Carlson Professor of Psychiatry
Division of Personality Studies
Department of Psychiatric Medicine
University of Virginia Health System

AUTHOR'S NOTE

FORWARD FROM THE MIND gives answers to questions you may have thought of before, and many answers to questions that you may *not* of thought of yet. If your heart is moved with compassion by the struggles you see around you and upon the earth, you have the ability to do everything you put your mind to. No longer will you suffer in silence and feel powerless to do anything about the illnesses, injustices and storms in and around you. The love placed within you is one way that you were made in the image of God – and with that, you are made to co-create with Him for manifesting changes in your life and the world. It is by recognizing and tapping into that Power and the unity of all at a quantum level, that the analytical brain needs to access the power of our spirit within the Divine Spirit. When this is realized, it changes everything, and all is possible! It is this that facilitates you to be a tool in the Hand of God. It is all there for you. It is all there for each one of us.

- A Fellow Worker for The Big Guy,
  Blessed Tiffany

CHAPTER 1

Space & Time is No Barrier in the Quantum World
Undeniable History of Mystics,
Healers & New Scientific Research

Do you want to live at that magical, lively and effervescent place between the candle and the flame? You can! Beneath the vast rippling surface of our consciousness lies an expansive world of quiet awareness where we live as co-creators in the holographic mind of the Cosmic Heart. This awareness is hard-wired into our very being, and in every culture in every part of the world, and in every period of time, history has shown man's *desire and ability* to access it. In many cases, only a fog-light of illumination has been visible through hundreds of years of misty fear and prejudice. Yet, man's passion for understanding beyond his own reality and into Divine space has propelled him eternally onward, and great discoveries in all fields have been awakened, and continue to be...

This book is for those who have already embarked upon their mystical journey; it is not for beginners on the path. The information here will expand and 'forward your mind' to remember how powerful you truly are as a spark from the One Flame. This journey has beckoned passionate adventurers for thousands of years, the knowing of *self,* that which is *beyond self,* and that which is purpose and *part of self.*

Where are you on your journey? Have you have rounded the bends and stumbled on rocks in the road, only to discover there are new facets of learning even while lying face-down? Have you traveled enough to discern what the destination looks like simply because you have a profound "knowing" about it in your very essence, no matter what others say? Forward movement occurs when we are not afraid to dance and play even on an unfamiliar trail, even when fear desires to stagnate and stop us.

In this book, you will learn of the power of Divine Connection. You will be taught an advanced process of distant healing where your spirit can go outside of your own physical body to heal another. You will learn methods to target the location of the person, find yourself in the room with them, see their surroundings, and watch and participate with God's energy in healing them.

You will also learn the deeper awareness of true spontaneous bilocation, where a person may physically manifest in more than one place at one time. And why it continues to be a common gift of adepts throughout the ages, and how you too can make yourself available for it. This book is an opportunity to move beyond mere human logic into a sphere of exploration where consciousness can shift effortlessly through real-time and other dimensions. Time does not move in a linear direction, and the choices we make here can ripple backward and forward. Would you like to manifest direct positive changes in your early life? What about manifesting positive changes in the history and future of the world?

Learn how SPI (specific prayerful intent) alters our quantum world and manifests changes in our reality and those of others by combining our intention with the cosmic strength of the "Great Observer," (the term often used in quantum mechanics for not using the word "God" or directly acknowledging same). See why and how medical intuition and "hidden" words of prophecy and knowledge are always readily available to us when we learn how to ask and access correctly. Find why a shift into higher awareness is often preceded by recognizing a defining moment our lives, and the different versions these may come in. Let me share with you my personal journey of expanding awareness and near-death experiences, and also what I am learning from my frequent episodes of stigmata, and spontaneous and miraculous healings and bilocation.

Seem fanciful stuff? Only if you ignore all physical evidence of years of research study, 100% of all eyewitness reports, and all the implications of quantum mechanics itself. In this day and time, there is much research available, and it is *not* because of lack of information that a person remains a skeptic; *but simply a lack of staying informed.*

"Energy is Eternal Delight" - English Romantic Poet William Blake

The mystic knows this passion. Whether cloistered as a religious, secluded in a guru's cave, or raising a family in the suburbs, the seeker explodes past the barriers. All preconceived boundaries fall aside in the fiery quest, with the common human becoming a powerful spiritual master as a by-product along the way.

The topics we will be discussing are also the deeper things of healing, a place where the average conversations between casual acquaintances dare not tread. Indeed, some topics might raise an eyebrow or two even amongst close friends! So let us come into this encounter with our minds cleared from prejudice, beyond any religion of habit, past bad metaphysics, and into a place of pure enlightenment as we seek an empirical experience of celestial reality in our life. Every true seeker is on a mystical path; a journey into spirituality and full awareness, past any constraints of space, time, and second-generation information.

"Mysticism avowedly deals with the individual not as he stands in relation to the civilization of his time, but as he stands in relation to truths that are timeless." - Mysticism by Evelyn Underhill

Often the seeker finds himself alone on any particular bend of his quest, with infrequent opportunities for intelligent discourse, new insights and experiences, or sharing notes. This book is your new companion and guide on this great journey. This book is *not* a parroting of familiar stories or an advertisement of branded techniques; choose another book for that - there are many available. But, this book strives to be more like a conversation with a new friend you meet along the road, one who has visited the destination before, and wishes to share with you what hotels are best, and which restaurants, attractions, etc. Their taste may not be your own, but it gives additional opportunities to pick and choose what is right for you. And a good guide also helps you develop some questions and strategy for yourself along the way.

I have put together a roadmap of sorts; one that will help you look at convergences and detours, possible short-cuts, and help with some "new construction" for the first-time traveler to these parts. For the experienced road warrior, there will also be intersections and several new "points of interest" and "scenic views" along the way. The true seeker does not fear when the soul ascends and descends through the mountainous hair-pin turns of the road. Often, a deep transformation process occurs only within these defining moments. They create an opportunity for understanding and awakening, as we learn to see different aspects of familiar things, or view aspects of entirely new ones.

It's a beautiful ride - and I invite you to take the top off your jeep and feel the warmth of the sun on your skin, and the wind in your hair. You are living in the explosion of the information age - and you are in the driver's seat with a state-of-the art electric cooler full of fruit and goodies next to you. That's me in the back, with my feet up - never mind me. I'm just going to close my eyes and "click out" for a moment to attend to some business back home - don't worry, I'll be right back - you're doing just fine. *This trip is going to show you more sights than you ever imagined! And it's fun too!*

"The most beautiful and most profound emotion we can experience is the sensation of the mystical. It is the sower of all true science. He to whom this emotion is a stranger, who can no longer wonder and stand rapt in awe, is as good as dead. To know that which is impenetrable to us really exists, manifesting itself as the highest wisdom and the most radiant beauty, which our dull faculties can comprehend only in their most primitive forms - this knowledge, this feeling is at the center of true religiousness." - The Universe and Dr. Einstein by Lincoln Barnett

There is No Substitute for Experience

On this journey, being intuitive is not a prerequisite to learning new things or to expand on previous ones. *But being curious is.* While some people seem to naturally have good results with one or more modalities, the majority of folk need to "awaken" to them and practice, practice, practice. In this book, there will be many reminders to do these things on your own.

Even for the "born natural," I have seen that practice increases the enjoyment and results of the chosen modality. I have seen great naturals stagnate

4

themselves and block many opportunities for advancement (pride in ability, fear of failure, etc.) and have seen the struggling student progress to greatness. Personal experience will teach you like no book or friend possibly can. I suggest you consistently spend a part of each day in experimenting with new things, which would be in addition to your book time - reading is not *having* an experience, but *preparing* you for one. Only empirical experience can satiate the mystic, fulfill the healer, and satisfy the scientist. So as you read this book, know that only *doing it* gets it done, and that is what gives you the *proof and ability needed to advance further.*

On Being Connected...Conscious and Unconscious Intention

We live on the same planet, breathe the same air, and drink the same nature-recycled water that our ancestors drank thousands of years ago. We are more affected by one another than we would like to believe. On the conscious side, we see TV programs about countries torn by disease and poverty and millions of children dying. We watch the news reports of continuing war causalities, tsunamis, beheadings, suicide bombers and flames engulfing buildings. Locally, we read the county newspaper about another missing child, another drug bust, another unsolved murder. On the home front, we try to figure out why our spouse is acting depressed, why Johnny was crying when he came home from school, why our boss is being such a hard-head, and if grandma is taking her medication. And, perhaps along the way, we ask ourselves why we have stomach pains and a headache...

Every physical cell in our being responds to the emotional reactions of the events we have processed and witnessed though the day, and this chemically and neurologically washes each cell and saturates our body. Many sensitive people find they have tremendously powerful reactions to stress, conflict, crowds and uncomfortable situations. Yet, when asked how we are doing, most of us will still automatically say, *"I'm fine."* And we may even believe it, since the conscious analytical brain *may or may not* feel that it has been influenced by any "outside" events at all.

Besides the physical impact, many of us do not fully realize the deeper subconscious level the events of the day have taken us to mentally.

5

Subconscious literally means *"beneath the threshold of consciousness, or that part of the mind that lies just below the level of conscious thinking."* If our subconscious has been programmed by fear and we live in a victim mentality, subconsciously we may still smell the twin billowing plumes of smoke rising from the Towers. Subconsciously, the starving child on TV is really our little Johnny lying helplessly in our arms. Subconsciously, fear tells us grandma dies; our spouse divorces us; we get fired; and all the gang murders, missing children and drug busts are in our own neighborhood. In fact, in the *very house next door!* This is dangerous, and as we advance in our awareness, we further see that our thoughts are actually intentions, which can greatly change our own reality for good or for evil.

Subconsciously we may also be repeating scenarios from our day, our past week, or our past year because of anger or guilt. Often we feel guilty because we didn't do anything about what "pushed our buttons" - we are *not* writing our senators, *not* organizing a neighborhood watch program, *not* finger-printing the county's children, *not* putting in the extra hours at work, yet also *not* spending more time with grandpa, *not* planning a romantic evening with our spouse, *not* playing more with little Susie, etc., etc. This produces a consciousness of guilt and powerlessness, coupled with a feeling of helplessness; *it seems that whatever we do is never good enough.*

This feeling can manifest either in our conscious mind or our subconscious one, and with it we usually throw in a taping of some traumatic childhood memories for good measure. Either way, we have enough menu items on the Guilt Platter to keep us insecure and stagnated for a long time, *as long as we choose to keep feeding off it.* The power of choosing our intention is the power of choosing the kind of life we want to lead.

Through time, people often become indifferent or desensitized about many things, at least on a surface level. We come to a point of overload, since we are taught such few ways of changing or relieving the situation. So, we place a barrier between us and the offending agent - and we start to shut out what is going on in the world, in our neighborhood, and even our own family. It's not as simple as "not caring." *It may be just the opposite.* But it seems like there's *nothing we can do.* But, are you creating it to be that way? Can you do something about it? Can you make your family, the neighborhood, or even the world, a better place from your own living room?

The "Oneness" of It All – Subatomic Soup

Living on earth encases us in a vibratory soup of subatomic particles - we are intrinsically linked together, *every part of us resonating with everything else.* But the connection we have goes much further than that - we emotionally "feel" subtle and tremendous inflections in our very soul. Slowly but steadily plodding along, science is now coming to the same conclusion that mystics have been saying throughout all time, namely, "we are all One."

French philosopher Rene Descartes, who became famous for saying *"Cogito ergo sum" ("I think therefore I am"),* attempted to put into words the human "sense of Self" of our conscious mind. We tend to "live in the brain," and this is the organ that gives us our sense of "reality," which is extracted from the filtered five senses that process our physical environment. This self-awareness also contributes to a feeling of separateness - our brain has masses of accumulated experiences that's at least slightly different from the combination of any one else on the planet, and we are extremely aware of this.

As our thinking matures, we find self-awareness can only go so far - we can't learn and experience all we want to by our self and through our own senses. So, when we become enlightened enough to make that decision to look beyond the filters of the ego Self, true wisdom can begin. It's at this point that we become receptive to "going out of our mind" (ha!) and can begin to accept "new realities" outside our own strictly physical senses.

From this point onward, the feeling of separateness disappears; *yet identity still remains, while becoming part of all other things.* You find yourself; you find Almighty God; you find all other living beings; and you *feel* them too. By letting go of "Self" you will gain everything. Now, a new saying comes to light, instead of "I think therefore I am," it is: *"we think therefore we are."* And in this awareness of Oneness, you find that many unusual and wonderful things here in the physical realm now reflect your Free Will connection with them…because you *are* them, and *your intention* influences it; it is simply an

7

extension of *your* physical, emotional and spiritual bodies.

The Zero Point Field

The Zero Point Field has discarded the isolationalism of Newtonian ideas, and brought us into the truth of the Universe: we are all connected with each other and the world around us. We live in a living ocean of microscopic vibrations, a collective consciousness of Light, a life force flowing through the universe, in the cosmic heart and breath of the Spirit of God. Everything is connected to everything else in a giant invisible web, and all of us are packets of energy constantly exchanging information with the giant life force of Divine Light himself. Living in this resonance of influence, this also means everything has an influence on us, and we have an influence on everything else as well.

To the spiritual person, whether she was born now or thousands of years ago, this information proves what has been witnessed and experienced all along. And now, far from the new physics destroying God, it has actually put Him back in the picture. Science now has the opportunity to be another tool for demonstrating all the things that it had previously turned its nose up on. Healing miracles, precognition, remote viewing, prayer - everything can now be re-examined by the skeptical analytical mind, and often what is found is all the needed statistics and numbers and "proof" in varying degrees, even with our often Dark Age prejudices. Even the "outer bounds" now deserves another look – for example, how group prayerful intention positively affects a polluted lake, and global environmental factors and weather patterns. There are never-ending opportunities to awaken.

Now, mankind has walked itself to the precipice of the cliff, and Spirit has timed it just right for there to be a further loosening of the veil over our ignorant eyes. Now we can dimly see where we are, what danger we are in, and can take the appropriate measures to come to an alertness of our missteps, and modify our course. But the *religion of science* has not let go so easily, and the *spiritual aspects of science* still continues to wager a struggle for financing and acceptance. An open mind is needed, and all preconceptions put aside. Once more we humans stand shoulder-to-shoulder at the dawn of a new creation, where we can choose to go beyond constriction and into

8

awareness, manifesting positive change at the awakening of this new paradigm. We are in this together, and we need to share with each other what we are seeing - the fog is lifting, so as in the beginning, let us echo: *"let there be light."* *(Gen.1:3)*

Individual Consciousness within Cosmic Thought – We Can Dance!

Look at the bee buzzing vibrantly in the middle of the hive, dancing 'in code' the directions to a new bountiful flower field and what delicacies have been found there. Soon tens, then hundreds or thousands of bees will join in with the vibrant dance. The workers confidently and eagerly lift off to bring home the new bounty. Hopefully the original worker bee chose wisely, and the harvest will be great, and the entire hive's chance for survival will be enhanced. He has danced the dance; the others chose to resonant with it; and together they benefit.

The bee had *individual consciousness within cosmic thought,* and that vibration literally stimulated a similar vibration ("entrainment") in all the others. All because of *one* bee - that brave soul who was seeking information down an unfamiliar path - fulfilled his in-born purpose to sweeten his world and share the information with others. And with that awareness of personal choice and power, comes individual life purpose.

Through personal application in my clinical practice, I have found time after time that no matter the condition of the physical health, *finding individual purpose is a central issue to sustained happiness.* We have a real need to feel that we are making a difference in the world. Just posing the questions: "Why am I here?" or "What is my purpose in life?" shows that we have a need for one. It gnaws at our inward parts; and we spend much of our lives throwing many things into this hole to try to fill the void. Nothing - not sex, materialism, fame, etc., affects much change for long. Nothing seems to move us beyond temporary gratification except the thing that created the need to begin with. We, just like the bees, have an in-born need to bring good things back to the hive, and sweeten our world, and we can't rest until we do. We have to share with others, and we have to dance!

9

With the gifts of out-of-body travel, local and distant healing, medical and psychic intuition and remote viewing, you have in front of you many opportunities for doing just that. There is no need to feel powerless any more. As we will see, you already have the right tools and many others hard-wired inside you. You only need to gain the confidence in how to use them, and in allowing the alignment and pulse of your particular beat to dance to the rhythm of the universe. Now, freedom will abound and every day can be filled with joy and happiness as you witness powerful changes around you. You will bask in the warm brilliance of fulfillment and satisfaction. No matter what may be going on in your life and in the world, there will never be anything that puts your fire out again - because the ember of knowing who you are, and what you can do, will glow forever true at your core. Certainly, in wielding these tools with confidence *nothing good is beyond your reach, for you have learned to dance.*

Being Unique in the Oneness of it All

Now, by opening to the modalities of bilocation, distant healing and remote viewing, it follows that attaining a higher secular education is not the only prerequisite for advanced helping of others. And, you won't need to wait in long airport terminal lines or take time off work to travel to exotic locations or to visit your relatives either. You won't need to worry about bodily harm in foreign countries. You can help heal people, animals, the environment, the world, all before rising for breakfast! Truly, nothing needs to be beyond your grasp, or even within the restrictions of the aspects of time. In your need to sweeten the world, you have found yourself living in the larger footprint of all the Ancient Masters, who in every culture have taken a form of the golden rule to heart: *"Love God with your whole heart, soul and mind...and your neighbor as yourself..."* (Mt. 22:37-39)

Without Passionate Intent, You will Fail

"Well," you might be thinking, *"that sounds too noble for me. I just want to have fun with these things!"* If that's the case, you need to find something else to do, because you will fail with these modalities. *Without a strong enough*

desire to cause an action outside of your own material body, you will not have enough power to do anything very well. You will be just sitting there, like a teapot on simmer, and never be able to go to the full rolling boil needed to do the real work, make the big differences, move your consciousness out of body, and have the great experiences. This is true for all things in life in which you want to be successful - you have to have a *real passion* for it to succeed, and that desire keeps you trying over and over again until it happens; *the passion makes it happen.*

Acknowledge the soul's need for making a difference, and bring this internal desire to a place of conscious command, to a full awareness of Mindful Intent. When you recognize this, you will succeed. With these advanced abilities, you must be focused. You must have one-pointedness of mind. You will find selfish intent, or just wanting to play around, won't be good enough to make much of an impact to do much of anything or go anywhere. You might as well stop right now, put down the book, and go watch paint dry.

We Can't Hide from the Vibrations Around Us

Now, let's look a bit further into what happened at the bee hive. And this time, instead of seeing ourselves as the scout who starts the dance, let's see ourselves as just another member of the hive. As more and more bees entrain and mimic the scout vibrations, the more quickly the dance vibrates throughout the hive, and there is limited ability to ignore it or to get out of its way. The vibration rushes through you, as a group member of the community, and soon you are also mimicking the dance. With bees, there is no choice, you cannot hide - it is part of your nature, you live in the hive. With humans, there is Free Will choice, and you can choose.

We have the choice to be the bee in the hive that starts the dance, or the one that vibrates to whatever rhythm is happening around us. How often have we come back from interaction with people and felt sad, lethargic and irritable? Ask yourself this question - are your vibrations lowering to the negative ones around you, is it possible that you are being entrained to someone else's chaotic emotional energy? Are you allowing a slowing and painful change of your personal dance, even adopting it as your own and forgetting the dance

11

you came in with? If you recognize this problem, recognizing it is the first step. The next step is *doing something about it.*

Living on earth intrinsically links all of us together in the hive. In this vibratory soup of subatomic particles, with every part of us resonating with everything else, we can see why it is so easy to feel overwhelmed - time is not linear - *we are picking up the dance from every single event around us, including the past.* Most of the time, this dance is of a very low vibration - not a happy, uplifting song - and we are being bombarded on all sides by it. It has familiar and consistent terminology the world over - it gives us the feeling of *being drained, under stress, depressed, tired all the time,* etc. But, when we make that conscious choice to rise to a higher vibration, we create a stronger ability for positive change, and the negative doesn't affect us nearly as much, or even at all. It is similar to the familiar psalm: *"Even though I walk through the valley of the shadow of death, I shall fear no evil..." (Ps. 23)* And this benefits the whole world, for we are sharing our sweet nectar, and fulfilling our life purpose.

So, we each have a choice in life. Either we can be a leader in the colony and start the dance - or we can simply be a member and take whatever vibes we are given. Which will it be? The choice is yours. Start the dance!

Superstrings and Quantum Mechanics

Einstein was motivated by passion. The last 30 years of his life was spent in relentless pursuit of a unified field theory - one that would illuminate the clear workings of the universe in simple and powerful principles. Many things were stacked against him, and in the last half century physicists have come a long way upon some wonderful foundations that Einstein laid. But even as the theories expound and change nearly every day, the sought-after level of insight into the deepest questions of the cosmos, the T.O.E or "Theory Of Everything" still hasn't been found. Perhaps science will find it in this generation, perhaps it won't. But, what has occurred - in lightning strike illumination - is full agreement on how much of what we thought we knew, *just doesn't work anymore!*

12

At this point, string theory is the only way we know to merge general relativity and quantum mechanics - but it also requires us to revise our concepts of space and time. Even the generally accepted number of dimensions in our universe (3 spatial and 1 time) has been convincingly overthrown by M-theory which involves 11 spacetime dimensions, and many physicists believe there are even more (... which there are).

"String theory declares that the stuff of all matter and all forces is the same...what appears to be different elementary particles are actually different "notes" on a fundamental string. The universe - being composed of an enormous number of these vibrating strings - is akin to a cosmic symphony...Every physical event, process, or occurrence in the universe is, at its most elementary level, describable in terms of forces acting between these elementary material constituents..." - The Elegant Universe by Brian Greene

This helps ease the analytical mind past many supposed barriers of what is real and what is *not* real and how everything is connected by an oscillation of resonance. So... you now have my permission to point your finger in the general direction of science and say *"but you can't prove out-of-body experiences (OOBEs), near-death experiences (NDEs), distant healing (DH), bilocation (BL) and remote viewing (RV) aren't real!"* Meanwhile, in your further awareness, you are journeying where average science wishes it could - well beyond the boundaries of space and time to experience firsthand many dimensions, spheres, and effects of energy/power/intent upon these various environments. In this state, you have become many things: a space traveler, a world explorer, an ancient shaman, and a highly realized spiritual being. You are truly becoming the full potential that your Maker created you to be.

The Stages of Awakening

Awakening comes in many stages, and is often initiated by a *defining moment* that pushes the envelope beyond our realms of understanding at that particular time. We have many subtle signals for advancement throughout the concentric circles of our life. For example, if we don't get the hint to step out of the dizzying and low-level repetition of events that manifest as frustration and

13

stagnation in our life, we trigger an escalation to bigger traumatic events. Many of these are manifestations of cause-and-effect of our poor choices. This might fit the definition of *going from bad to worse.* It also fits the Type A attitude who ignores their mental, spiritual or physical health and ends up being susceptible to tumors, diseases, and emotional disorders of all kinds. It is often the rawness of the deepest part of our soul telling us to "wake up!" "pay attention!" "slow down!" "be gentle!"

Most of the time, an enlightened person can tell you the *very moment* they awoke. For example, a cancer patient may use surgery, radiation and chemotherapy with her choice of strictly conventional medicine until the doctor tells her: *"all we can do is give you more morphine - go home and say your goodbyes - there's nothing more we can do."* The doctor's conventional conclusions are often a combination of statistics and terminology that stimulates the patient to fear and to shut down any hope of getting well. But, the patient doesn't have to resonate to that negative vibration in the hive if she doesn't want to. She can make another Free Will conscious choice…and at that moment she makes the decision to go beyond the original format, and open to new ideas. This might include practicing visualization, herbs, prayer, various forms of energy medicine; or perhaps even that healer in California she was told about several months ago…

At That Moment, Everything Changes

(1). A man pops a few more aspirin into his mouth and blindly stares out from behind his piled-high desk of papers which he has no hope to finish. Intently he thinks about his wife and the love-making of that morning - and at that moment immediately finds himself at home in his hall way, more real than any dream. He sees his wife startle, look in his direction, and make eye contact with him from her chair in the living room. She gasps and actually thinks she sees her husband - she certainly felt his presence - and for a brief moment he could see her too. Instantly popping back to the office, he excitedly calls his wife, who surprisingly and happily confirms the visit. *How is this possible to see through distance and space, with one consciousness recognizing the other?*

14

(2). A homemaker picks up the newspaper and reads about a boy missing since yesterday. Emotionally moved, she puts her hand lovingly over his picture and wishes she knew where he was. Immediately, a vision of the boy tied up in a locked building adjacent to the local city park appears in her mind's eye - and at that moment she knows she will never be the same. She reaches for the phone to call the police. Her mind floods with more details. She doesn't know how she'll explain where she got the information, but she knows without a doubt that what she saw was real and important. *How could she be seeing this missing child and have such details about it?*

(3). A sad and broken woman gets struck by lightning, has a near-death experience (NDE), and comes face-to-face with the other side, where Jesus connects her with the ability to be a gifted healer and intuitive. The experience shakes her strict denominational little world - and at that moment her mind opens, and she realizes most of everything she had previously learned was false or only partly true. She spends the rest of her years processing the new things she has learned, has a second NDE, stigmata, and fully utilizes the celestial "keys" left in the door…as she writes and heals and shares the new information with anyone who will listen. Yes, this is I. *How does one heal, inspire and connect the true potential of every heart to the pulse of the Divine Heart beating within them?*

It is in these moments that heaven and earth kiss – they are examples of being that place between the candle and the flame, and with it, a fertile swelling of transcendental information births new glorious and fruitful children. The reality of true self oscillates between every degree of lucidity and shade of consciousness, and the ego lets go of any need for separateness, fear or selfishness. And along the way, each of us discovers a few things: we don't die when our body does; time isn't a straight line moving only forward; our consciousness can be separated purposefully from our living bodies and rejoined again at will. We learn that one body's physical health can be affected by another body's invisible energetic one; our Divine connection is real and has a Personality and Persona; we have a direct influence on all things that have ever been or ever will be; and we co-create with our pure and Holy intentions in that place of high vibration and Free Will within the Cosmic Heart of God.

The illumination of self, and the Absolute self, is a stage of growth that is often called the World of Becoming, or the "Illuminative Way." *(ibid.* Underhill) It is in this place that we recognize the effort of the mind to bridge the illusionary gap between Creator and Creation, and the soul accepts the challenge of weighing discernable truth to that of simple imaginative phenomena. Now the quest deepens for the mystic traveler, as only empirical experience and practice will answer what she needs to know, at a level that her soul will accept, remember, and acknowledge.

CHAPTER 2

Becoming Stronger in the Broken Places
Breaking Through the Barriers of Fear

The human spirit is constantly in a state of emergence from the darkened cave of illusion. So many things that we thought were true and sure in ancient times (such as the blood ebbing and flowing like a tide in the body, instead of circulating) were just our limited perception through smoke and mirrors. We are on a never-ending, always changing, cosmic pilgrimage. This journey, which of necessity encompasses overwhelming soul importance and significance, can overly stimulate the advancing traveler. As a friend accompanying you, please let me interject a word of caution here - balance is needed in all things.

You still own a physical body here, one that needs to work, eat, sleep, be taken for walks and produce excrement. You still have relationships to nurture, and responsibilities to take care of. There are many things in this book that will require time and practice, and conscious intention of spirit connecting to Spirit for incredible, beyond-the-body activities. But, *you cannot live entirely outside of your body all the time.* It is unhealthy on all levels: physically, emotionally and spiritually, I know - I speak from experience! As with any regiment for health, consistency and moderation is needed. Just as it's better to eat several small meals a day instead of just one big one, so it is with buying out a multitude of small allotments of time to develop these important supernatural gifts, instead of trying to master it all in a two-week vacation.

Grounding and Balance Needed When Learning to Fly

Inside of me there is a secret place that I always have to find balance and peace with - a strong desire to leave everything and everybody, to go find a place of absolute solitude, and be out-of-body and in-connection all the time. I dream of having a secluded place on a mountain somewhere, a place where I can fast, fully discard the illusion of the veil, and sustain full union with

Source…even until there is no body to come back to. The very real stimuli for me are my unforgettable near-death experiences, and stigmata, which all overwhelm me with a Love so deep and effervescent that I am perpetually *homesick* all the time. It is that Love and promise I gave to the One of All Love, that keeps me here, because I know the importance of the work to be done and the need to finish it. He also reminds me of the joys of this physical life as the gold is shared and experienced by others. And *you* have important work to do too, and are encouraged to share the gold and see the joys as well.

In the beginning of my journey, it was difficult to find any kind of balance between my spiritual life and my physical needs. My daughter would often call me up to ask, "Mom, did you eat today?" She knew I would forget, since it was not important to me, and neither was sleep. But, it is important to be a satisfactory care-giver while we are in the body. It is a wonderful tool for everything we need to accomplish here, and we need to respect it and treat it as a temple; a place that holds sacred knowledge and spiritual flame, and honor it as such.

There are wonderful by-products of the healing work for me, including that I have not had a single day of sickness (beyond some sniffles) since the lightning strike, which was my first near-death experience. And with the added regeneration that occurs during stigmata, I also look about ten years younger than most women my age; and I'm stronger and have more endurance and energy than many people, male or female. Most people have a difficult time believing I have four grown children, two of whom have been married for several years, and that I am a grandmother. I even plan on birthing a couple more children of my own, since I am more than capable and love the little ones and interaction of family life.

Consistently tapping into the stream of Spirit keeps you refreshed, vibrant and vital in mind and body. It is a place of timelessness and connection beyond the restraints of perceived physical limitations or year of birth. And indeed, we are not walking this journey on our own energy, but are part of the whole, and all the energy is there to sustain us. It is not only about giving, but receiving, and it is all there for us, and that includes you too!

18

Your Conduit of Healing Can Advance and Change Too

There are many times during a healing I can barely hold on with the amount of current pulsating through and around my body. The strong vibrations start at my head, run down my body and through and out my hands and down through the soles of my feet to the earth. This invisible current creates outward visible effects in all things around me, seen and unseen. Consistently the lights at the Institute surge or go off, the computer screens run purple streaks across them, the lobby TV/video presentation flickers or goes off, the credit card machine won't work, etc. Also the heat in the healing rooms raises noticeably many degrees, and the music turns up or goes off. I understand that there is power here beyond my own, and so does the person under my hands, for they experience it in their own bodies and minds, and have an empirical experience with God on their own. I just happen to be in the room.

I create an opportunity to go direct, I have complete faith without restraint or doubt, there is nothing to clog up the channel. I then get myself out of the way, and allow the person's Free Will to receive what they are asking for, and supernatural events and miracles manifest. It is not something I am doing to someone, for it is a three-way connection of intention, giving, and receiving. So as a receiver, the client has an active part in participation of his healing. It is like God is the electrical powerhouse; I get to be an extension cord for a while, and the client on the table is the lamp. They can choose to turn it up and receive a little and the bulb will only glow – or they can choose to really crank it up and receive a lot and the lamp will burn strong and brightly!

My job is to believe all miracles are available at all times; if I didn't little would happen and I would be out of a job! I stand beside the client in full faith and expectation. Truly, time and time again I have seen that nothing is held back from us, The Big Guy never just gives crumbs. But often it is the client's own stuff (unworthiness issues, etc.) that can clog the receiving channel, so the more we can open, the more we can absolutely expect miracles. And in this wondrous life, we never have to do it alone, so someone who encourages self-care and worthiness can literally be a God-send, to remind each one of us how loved we already are.

19

Compassion is the Catalyst to Heal

Since my last NDE where I visited in the Oneness with Christ, and during the most strenuous cases for healing (i.e., cancer, AIDS) I feel burning pain in the very center of my hands, and the same in the center of my feet, and in my right side. As time has gone on, these places of burning began to blister, and to open up and bleed. Now, very consistently (almost every month, for three to five days at a time) I experience what is called stigmata, or "the wounds of Christ." It comes with visions of the past, and of the future. It comes with a clarity of being and unity with the Oneness of God, in a way that I experience at no other time. This is a place where all knowledge is there for me, even while holding onto a body. The Spirit of Christ lets me know that He is communing with me. It is an overlay of Spirit, me experiencing Him, and Him experiencing me.

This is a trueness that I wish to share with you – light and dark can't be in the same place together, so the brighter and lighter we are, the more God can experience life through us. The truest sense of communion, sharing and Oneness occurs in this place of surrender and trust. There is strength in vulnerability. There are no limitations on how unique and wonderful our lives may become when we finally surrender all things, for we gain everything and have lost nothing but fear. It the place all things manifest.

When doing the healings, even hundreds of them at conventions, *I am not drained by the work,* though I often feel I've been in a Jacuzzi too long. I feel the ecstasy of joy in my heart, beyond the meaning of words. How the healings feel to the client, and how the Connection flows in your body either in personal hands-on or by distant healing, will be unique for each situation. I live in the Christ connection, and have been met by Him at both my NDEs, I greatly respect and recognize the grace Father has placed before all mankind, but recognize also that The Big Guy manifests Himself to His kids in many ways. I also know that there are many healers, and their healings don't have to be the same as mine to be very good healings.

20

We are not here in comparison to anyone else, but each striving to consistently advance ourselves spiritually, emotionally and physically. We all have different and personally unique ways to connect, but we are all His kids, and brothers and sisters to each other.

At the Institute, where I may see someone for an hour, I never feel the client's pain in my own body, unless I ask for it to get a better picture of what is going on. If medical intuition is requested and I am having difficulty interpreting what I am seeing on my internal visual screen, feeling what they feel gives me a new perspective. But I am careful not to do this for very long, because it can be difficult to shake off. The human mind and body is made to be very empathetic to one another, and this can lead to not knowing what is *mine* and what is *yours*. I suggest you make the intention of using this method only periodically. At the conventions, there may be 30 seconds or less for a healing, and I spend more time with my spirit half-out of the body than fully in, being in a totally surrendered state to allow full connection. Most people faint and fall from the blissful surge of the Divine Spirit they feel at the touch of my hand, while others get healed while still sitting in the audience.

I have people to help catch those who are falling and bring them gently to the floor, where God continues to work with them. Each one is given unique experiences, visions, wisdom, visits from departed loved ones, words from Father, or physical, emotional and/or spiritual healings. With each one, I receive a healing too. For days afterward I feel like I need 20# of lead in my shoes to keep me from floating up from the ground and into the blissful sky! It is a joyful feeling of elation, and just like the healings the clients receive, it has a beautiful ripple effect in all areas of my life.

As you come more fully into the mystical life, your sleep patterns may change too. For a long time I needed no more than 3 or 4 hours of sleep per night - compared to 8-10 hours previously. Now since the stigmata, that fluctuates, depending on how I am maintaining balance in my physical, emotional and spiritual life. It affects my recuperation time.

When I "click-out" of body, I find that being out-of-body or astral allows the physical home body to rest; *but the spirit still needs adequate time to rest as*

21

well. It is important that you still allow your consciousness to play for a few hours or so; to allow processing of data. Perhaps watch a movie, or play a video game. Also, since most people notice that their physical body seems to stay in one position while they are *out*, there may be an amount of physical soreness that needs to be worked out of the muscles and joints, which would have happened by normal movement, stretching and turning during regular sleep. All these things are tidbits I am sharing with you, and you can choose to nibble on them now, or save them for later, but you will need this food to nourish you along the journey, or else you will tire out and need an extended period of rest before continuing on the trail, for you are blazing new frontiers.

The New Pioneer

The brave American pioneers headed westward in canvas wagons, and often their only instruction manuals were *The Farmer's Almanac* and the *Holy Bible.* The smarter ones also gleaned what they could from others they met along the way, listening to all the information available, and weighed this against reason and personal experience. Whatever situation they ran into, they tried to adapt to or maneuver around, always with their goals set passionately in front of them. And wild animals attacked them, land battles were fought, weather destroyed, disease marauded, and famine struck. And the pioneer spirit kept renewing itself, and the west was settled, one acre and one goal at a time.

As we got into space exploration, the same renewal of spirit and passion motivated mankind to even greater (literal) heights. The western pioneer rarely dreamed of manned flight, since all he saw was a covered wagon and wooden wheels sitting firmly on the ground. Most folk were limited in their concept of what was possible. But, there were the occasional dreamers as well, and these are the ones that broke the barriers in mind and thought. Now, we stand upon a new horizon, the exploration of *inner space* - and the drive must be the same. Will you restrain yourself to see only see what is in front of you, and not also what *is* to be seen?

"Man is in the process of changing, to forms that are not of this world; grows he in time to the formless, a plane on the cycle above. Know ye, ye

22

must become formless before ye are one with the light." - The Emerald Tablets of Thoth

It takes determination and bravery to head out on this new pattern of thought, since the wind will blow (people will talk), church steeples fall (some religions will try to hinder you), and famine will cover the land (you will go through plateaus where nothing seems to be happening). And at each one of these occurrences, you will have new decisions to move ahead, step backwards, or stay still. You have the choice to quit at any time; and you can stake your claim right where you are, at any given moment. But just be sure you are choosing your steps - or lack of them - for the right reasons, since this is *your personal soul journey*, and no one else should be interfering with such intimate decisions. Why limit yourself without even trying? Why stay alongside the road when the road continues on to so many interesting places?

"The Force is strong with this one, it is..." - Yoda, *The Star Wars Trilogy*

Believe me, if you let *someone else* tell you what to do, manipulating your Free Will choices about these very personal things, *this is what will happen:*

(1). You will regret it later.
(2). You will resent the power this person has over you.
(3). You will be angry at yourself for allowing manipulation to occur.

If you don't want to allow your physical body to be flooded with random vibrations that may be around you, it's time for you to set the pace and dance the dance. Even if you sit out one of the dances, YOU are the one who should decide when and where. Don't let anyone else try to tell you what only your own heart and soul knows for sure. *Don't give your power away,* this is a journey where you are creating empirical experiences as you go.

Fear of the unknown is one of those things that keep us hanging tight to our body. To be successful in exploring this new frontier, *you must let go of fear.* For me, the only way is through complete surrender and trust in the Divine One. I never feel I am *leaving* anywhere, but *going to.* Yet in many ways, there really is no coming or going at all, but simply a movement of intention,

23

of openness, of embracing. Like a fish in the ocean that doesn't know what water is, how oxygen intake happens or propulsion works, yet still thrives, so are we in our subatomic particles swimming happily away. And, being a little smarter than fish, we get to solve some of the Big Questions and have the Big Adventures along the way.

Breaking through the Barriers of Fear

"The spirit is an area of growth most of us set aside, half hoping the day will come when some soul-stretching peak experience will lift us out of our ordinary consciousness for a glimpse of the sacred and eternal. But we have to prepare for taking such a path. We need to change the way we measure time and to relax our insistence on control...The present never ages. Each moment is like a snowflake, unique, unspoiled...and can be appreciated in its surprisingness...If every day is an awakening, you will never grow old. You will just keep growing." - New Passages by Gail Sheehy

We are *never too old* to learn and experience new things; in fact, it is this attitude that keeps us young. I have seen teenagers with the motivation of a 70 year old man; and 70 year old men jogging and going to night school! Time seems to move more swiftly as we age, but the spirit has timeless abilities. And this, in turn, affects how we view today. Each day is an opportunity for new skills when we live beyond fear, and journey toward knowledge and perfection in love and light.

"God is love. Whoever lives in love lives in God, and God in him...there is no fear in love. But perfect love drives out fear, because fear has to do with punishment. The one who fears is not made perfect in love." (1 Jn. 4:16-18)

It is natural to be hesitant when you step onto an unknown path. But keep in mind that you share with the Universal Mind, and are made in the image of the Creator - which also means that you are built for exploration and re-creation. We know that anything worth doing is worth doing well, but it is rarely easy. Replacing fear with mature love is a constant human endeavor - we have been inundated with scare tactics and threats of punishment throughout our entire lives. There may be times you are timid to take the next step and are afraid. If you are, then step forward anyway and *do it afraid* - don't let fear stagnate you, or take away the peace and deeper wisdom you were created to appreciate and enjoy. It is your birthright as a beloved child of God.

"If the universe is based on energy and attraction, this means that everything is vibrating to particular frequencies. When the frequency with which you're vibrating is in contradiction with the frequency of the universal supply, you create a resistance, thereby inhibiting that flow of abundance into your life space. Your individual vibrations are the key to understanding the art of allowing...remember, it's always about being in harmony with your Source. Your thoughts can either emerge from a beingness that's in rapport with intention or in contradiction with it." - The Power of Intention by Dr. Wayne Dyer

The "monkey mind" of activity will think up all kinds of things to distract you from your goals. But you are the one in charge of what you want to do. *You are in control of your actions.* Think of the opportunities placed in front of the one who walks *beyond restraint* - so much is possible, and can be done, has been done, and *IS* being done! By incorporating these modalities into your lifestyle, you will be setting the rhythm for those around you, and the world will hum happily to your song.

The Need is Great – the Opportunities Immeasurable

We need more local and distant healers, and intuitives: Asia, South America, China, South Dakota - no matter where in the world you are, you can be facilitated for healing and comforting the sick and impoverished, war torn, diseased and broken. You can be at a grandmother's bedside releasing fear of death and easing her spirit into loving transition by inspired words and hands-on healing. You can aid in finding unknown or undiagnosable medical conditions in an ailing child through medical intuition. You can be a connection and messenger of hope and love to those who are mourning for loved ones who have transitioned in death. You can balance and empower the emotional state of thousands, helping to lift depression and anxiety by an infusion of Divine vibration of the highest frequencies. You were created with many natural gifts, and can choose to tap into the Supernatural ones as well.

25

There are endless opportunities to use these abilities for good.

We need more remote viewers and prayer warriors: since nothing is hidden from your eyes, you can aid world peace-keeping and help identify areas and persons who try to conceal weapons of mass destruction, and manifest change through specific prayerful intention. You can help find missing children before they expire from the elements, or before an abductor gets away with murder. You can check on your mother-in-law to see if she got on the plane, and the children off to school. You can look at time in the future or past, as an aid to possible earthquake zones or places of catastrophe. You can make astounding maps for space exploration or for focusing information collection for satellites. You can help find artifacts in the Egyptian sand or buried shipwrecks on the ocean floor. Nothing is beyond your capability when you realize the Source and river of connection between all things, and bathe in that deep refreshing water. Take a dip!

Become the True Potential You Were Created to Be

Everything is speeding up now - today human consciousness is evolving very quickly, and important choices are being made. Those in the Light are shining brighter, and those in the darkness are growing darker still. But the day is dawning, and Light will win. There are many who are needing your brightness to light the way right now, to feel the glow of your happiness resonate and dance within them and to remember who they are. They have been filled and immersed in lower vibrations for a long time now, and have often forgotten the warmth of the light on their face, and the effervescent bliss emanating from their hearts. Their candle is glowing low, and in some cases has even gone out.

With these gifts available and used by you, you are brought into the realm of the *mystic: "one whose truth stems solely from divine revelation."* This is the highest form of human consciousness…soul recognizing truth by the remembrance and raw emotion it stirs, and the ego it kills. Strictly traditional thinkers, atheists, or the spiritually timid are forewarned that the material presented within these pages may rock their world - and a new foundation will call out to be built, as the old one tumbles down. But those who are serious in seeking the truth of "I AM" will find the true reality that God allows for, and indeed, has always encouraged - empirical experience. And that is the opportunity you can gain here; use these words as a touch-stone for what you can do, by reading about what I and others have done and are doing. It is the way mankind has advanced true conscious awareness throughout the existence of time - first-hand experience and personal evidence.

"The absolute subjectivity of revealed truth precludes all considerations or uncertainties which stem only from the ego. When the ego collapses, all argument ceases and is replaced by silence. Doubt is the ego. One could say that the ego is primarily a complex doubt structure that keeps itself rolling on my manufacturing endless, unsolvable problems, questions, and distractions. When confronted by the overwhelming certainty of Absolute Truth as it is reflected from the Self, the ego collapses and literally dies. That is the only real death possible, and only the illusory self is vulnerable to it." - I, Reality and Subjectivity by David R. Hawkins, M.D., Ph.D.

Interpretation, Translation and Misinformation

Translation of spiritual visions into material words caused interpreter problems in the past, and still does today! The constant bantering among denominations over the Bible books of Revelation, Ezekiel and Jeremiah (to name a few) underscores this. Division has occurred throughout all religions and regions, underscoring the strange twists and turns of human interpretation. Often getting bottle-necked and closed up somewhere along the way, hard-sought wisdom can go unheard; even when there are eager ears to hear it.

How many misunderstandings occur between you and your mate on a week-to-week or even day-to-day basis? Now, in our imagination, let's separate the both of you - let's say your work has necessitated you to live on opposite coasts for a while. You initially think everything will be fine - you have each other's love letters, and you try to talk on the phone everyday. Short-term, the relationship may do OK, but over a period of time, *it will fall apart.* No doubt you have seen in your own life that a critical factor to normal development and deepening of a healthy relationship is constant communication. If you don't, you will find difficulty with getting even the smallest thought across, so much common groundwork has failed to be made, and the personal and relationship foundations create cracks and stagger from weakness. Without communication, it is as if you and your mate are coming from two different worlds now - and many marriages fail on that note.

Now, on an imaginary earth-wide scale, take away the email and cell phones; multiply distance by mountain ranges, rivers, oceans, weather and tribal battle lines; throw in historic cultural and skin differences; add different dialects and languages (which may not even have a translation for the word you want to say); and, ooh yes, *thousands of years of separation.* I would say the chances are pretty good that the relationship is going to suffer. This is the relationship that we have as we approach a relationship with God through only traditional means.

So what about religion? It was one of the first questions I asked after my connection with Him. I asked, "which religion is the right one?" And He said: "ALL THOSE WHO LOVE ME." This reply is just like Him, to answer everything and nothing at the same time! Later, I asked about the Holy Bible, was it accurate? The answer: "ALL HOLY BOOKS ARE INCOMPLETE, SO THAT MAN MAY REACH OUT FOR ME, AND I WILL REVEAL MYSELF. AND THEY WILL EACH KNOW ME AND I WILL GREET THEM." He desires us to each have an empirical experience, to have a personal relationship and reveal Himself to each one of us. I would say that also shuts down anyone stating they have a "corner on the market" by exclaiming they are the only ones with true knowledge. Like a good Dad, Father desires *all* His kids to crawl up on His lap – all of them!

Building Blocks of *Knowing*

I see that wisdom is available to anyone, in any period of time, in any place in the world. And I have no problem in recognizing that Godly intervention can choose to protect the most valuable insights, often has, and still does, so it can walk unimpeded throughout history. After all, we have seen that mankind has been consistently raising his frequency over time, and especially so now - so something must be *sticking.* But, how many people still live only within social

28

presumptions and accept misunderstandings as truth? Here, again, lies the beauty of learning to access and use these Godly Supernatural modalities for yourself. Once you have begun to experience a few things, you will be able to better interpret the original language of old as *written upon your very soul.*

And – sorry for this - but you *still* won't be able to explain it very well to anybody! At least, not in a way that truly encompasses the visions you will see and feel. The average person feels so isolated and separated from God that the possibility that One can be personally known and experienced seems just too unbelievable. How do you describe a personal immersion of light and infinite love that has no beginning, no end, and has a central location but is also in everything and not separate from anything? How do you explain the death feeling of being a single raindrop falling into the sea, and instead of losing your own identity in the blending, you become greater and larger than anything you ever felt before, and live through all things? And then the expansion of that raindrop rippling out, only to discover the ocean is a raindrop as well? How do you describe touching *the very face of God?*

If you truly *knew* that your spirit survives outside of the human body - *that you never really die,* how would it affect how you are living your life every day? Just from this building block alone, immense changes would ripple throughout your life. How you look at your religion, how you interact with people overwhelmed with health problems, what goals you have set for yourself, what time means to you, how you act at funerals and what you say to grieving friends, etc. Everything would be changed. Everything would need to be re-thought, with new actions and interactions.

Now, what if you added another block of *knowing* upon this one; how would it change your life if you saw spirits on the other side waiting to be born. Whew - now we have a whole new mix, more things to figure out and how they fit into the parameters of what you thought you knew. Is this reincarnation? Or is this the real meaning of *anastasis* (Greek) "raising up, standing up," of *resurrection of the dead?* Could this be first-time or original creation? Are these simply thought-forms of group memory? Is this just a glimpse of the cloth of time ripping through a non-linear dimension? You can easily see how many more questions will be raised by the answers you

29

personally find, and the ability to have answers will give you more questions.
It is a very compelling journey! And you will be sure to seek, and find, many
more answers along the way.

The Life of Miracles

As this unfolding, blossoming and foundation building continues, many
wonderful things beyond ordinary comprehension are going to follow. Perhaps
healing miracles will occur spontaneously in your presence, or you may attract
highly realized humans to bilocate to you for a chat, or you to them. Perhaps
you will have precognition of a destructive event and also be able to lessen or
transform its duration or intensity through intention and prayer. Many events
you will experience are going to fall outside of the subjects of this particular
roadmap, but you will surely be compelled to keep on driving. When that
happens, I have succeeded in my goal - after all, spiritual awareness toward
Divine Love is not a destination, but a journey, and it never ends. Who would
want it to?

As you continue developing intuition and abilities, you will also be able to
recognize the similarities between them, and the important differences. Such
it is with distant healing and remote viewing. Let's look at them now, and the
importance of laying a good foundation, and establishing a resonance between
client and healer.

CHAPTER 3

Establishing Healer/Client Resonance
"Cell Memory," the Five Senses, and the Holographic Brain

One of the most interesting concepts of quantum mechanics has been this discovery: that what we assume to be reality is profoundly affected by the mere fact of human observation. Let's look at a few more concepts. *Superposition* is where a quantum particle can be in a combination of two or more states at the same time. Identical photons create an interference pattern before observation - and then (when observed) the wave suddenly turns into particle! Also, with quantum *spin,* all electrons are noted as spinning in different directions, until (when observed) *a direction is somehow specified,* and they start to spin in only one direction! As Neils Bohr stated; *"Anyone who is not shocked by quantum theory has not understood it."*

It is only when the atom is being watched that it remains as a particle - when the atom is not being watched, it reverts back to a waveform. So we have proof that light is both wave and particle, but according to quantum mechanics, we can't truly consider it to be either until we look at it. *Entanglement,* (sometimes called *nonlocality)* is where a *faster-than-the-speed-of-light* signal is instantaneously communicated between two particles which somehow remain in touch with each other no matter how far apart they are. What happens to one instantly happens to the other, even across a galaxy, through this entangled waveform connection. And if we look at the beginning of the universe through a "Big Bang" theory, we see all energy (which includes us) was entangled in the very beginning, so we all have an indent with each other now, even though we may be far apart. Very simply, what one of us does, does *affect all others.*

"What is not in doubt is that there has to be some kind of nonlocal communication taking place that instantaneously informs the undisturbed particle of the type of measurement we have just carried out on its partner." - Quantum by Jim Al-Khalili

The Power of Focused Observation – Manifesting Change by Brain or Spirit

We are highlighting the power of observation, and the inherent life of all things in the Whole. By merely giving attention, physicists are noting change takes place in the primary structure of the building blocks of the universe. Now take this *power of observation by a man of flesh,* and add a bit more wood to the fire - use the *power of intention by added willful connection of the shared intention of the Whole, of God Himself.* What do we have? What do you think could happen? Does it make sense that there might be more changes realized through intentionally desiring a willful outcome, rather than just observing one? Could this be the "God-Spot" where prayer manifests miracles, where the physical body bilocates, where levitation happens and multiplication of foods occur? What happens when highly focused intention is turned to these subatomic levels? This is where the reality of Supernatural events occur, and changes manifest in the blink of an eye, in the Eye of God.

Much of what is being observed in the field of quantum mechanics is still not fully understood by science. And much of what we are experiencing as mystics and spiritual masters cannot be proven scientifically. The "Theory of Everything" still has not been realized. But, the *effects* are there - physicists are just trying to find *the middle of the alphabet.* They have seen the beginning and understand some of the letters toward the end - now they have to logically figure out how one gets to the other. How many more surprises wait in the journey between A and Z? As we have seen, only those emerging from the dark cave of illusion will stretch their mind *forward* to find out! Will you be one of these?

The Resonance Between All Things

"Dust as we are, the immortal spirit grows like harmony in music; there is a dark inscrutable workmanship that reconciles discordant elements, makes them cling together in one society." - William Wordsworth

I would like to take a further look at *nonlocality* and how we might see applications to life around us in a mystical sense. As we have seen, this

32

entanglement happens when signal is instantaneously communicated between two objects, no matter how far apart they are, because they have been together before. I see this as not much different than what we might call *resonance*, which is a transfer of energy from one system to another. In our macro (large) world, we see that when two systems are oscillating at different frequencies, this resonance occurs until *entrainment* occurs, where both systems vibrate at the same rate. We see this in "life-less" inanimate objects as well as fully biological systems, such as the human body. This shouldn't come as any surprise, since everything has atoms as the common denominator.

Entrainment in group settings: It has long been noted in women's dormitories and other places where ladies are grouped together, that within a short amount of time all the menstrual cycles of the women will coordinate to occur at the same time. Also, scientists have found that disembodied animal hearts left close together in a lab will start beating the same rhythm. And how many times have you heard the neighborhood frogs sounding out in unison? What about the crickets? Now, does entrainment occur with the group effect of panic in a stadium, or depression in an office setting, or excitement at a concert? There is no reason to think this would be any different. All things oscillate to the frequencies around them. Remember the bee in the hive?

Think about it - how many times have you felt very strong emotions without being actively aware of the source? Doesn't this fit right in with our common language, such as the statement: "just being around him is so depressing," or "I feel happy just being there," or even "we get along so well - it seems like we're on the same wave-length!" Yes, there is physiology involved too - but since we now know about nonlocality, where do we actually draw the line? Hmmm, OK, now add another piece to this puzzle - when your mother calls you up because she feels "something is wrong." When she lives a thousand miles away and somehow feels something happening to you, wouldn't you say that's an example of the direct effect of quantum nonlocality? It doesn't take an intuitive to do this. It is part and parcel of living on the planet, and living in the rhythm of the Cosmic Heart. We just don't normally realize it, or choose to access it on purpose, although we can. And as the case with mom, *love* is a motivating factor to this power.

Tapping into the Highest Energy Transfer –
Healing as a Function of Entrainment

See how easy it is to take the next step of atomic interaction and understand the Oneness that governs all things? Does this give you more of a reason to understand how distant healing, remote viewing, and indeed, all intuitive gifts operate? Might healing be a way of entrainment as we are facilitated to raise the vibrational frequency of an injured or an imbalanced body up to a place of wholeness and resonance? Now how much further can it go when the healer taps into the Oneness of the Universe for the energy transfer? Can a high frequency human become so fully connected that the oscillation between the Divine Mind and human mind can operate in immediate and spontaneous nonlocal entrainment, and any intention immediately become manifested fact? YES! Could this be a possible explanation to where it is said *"the kingdom of God is within you?"* (Lk. 17:21) All things are possible, and manifestation of healing miracles and other supernatural changes in and beyond our environment occur every day for those minds in full Connection, unclouded by fear or doubt.

"The functional state of a living being depends on the frequencies that can be two aspects: strong or weak, and concentric or disorderly. A strong concentric thought field corresponds to a special function or a Qigong state for a person. From this, various parapsychical phenomena may be explained. The thought field is possibly a model unifying different paranormal biological phenomena, and is a bridge between religion and natural science." – Y-Fang Chang, *The Journal of Religion and Psychical Research,* pg 191, 2004

Entrainment in Nonliving Things

If you step into a music store and strike a bass key on a piano (preferably a low note since the oscillation is slower and more dramatic to the human ear), the un-touched guitar hanging on the wall next to it is also going to resonate that tone. As a musician, I can attest you will hear the drone of untouched violins and mandolins humming along too! When I operated my recording studio in Tennessee, we had to make sure that no other wood-bodied instruments were in the room when we were recording. The additional tone could be heard in the headphones. Instruments made of other, harder elements such as silver or brass didn't seem to be affected as much; if only because it was at a frequency that was out of our conscious hearing level. This is an example of entrainment in nonliving things.

In college I took a fun class on music therapy. Although it's not often recognized in the west, music or sound therapy has a history that goes back thousands of years. In many cases, these therapies are integral to certain healing or spiritual modalities, and the basic desire is for the client to be brought beneficial frequencies of the music being used.

Once, I had the unique experience of standing on a raised platform underneath a huge cylinder-shaped bell in a courtyard in Hawaii, while a wooden beam was released into the side of it, directly over my head. Once was all I needed! I not only *heard* the vibes, but *felt* them rippling all throughout my body. It was a pleasant sound, and an extraordinary feeling. I certainly felt "entrained" for several hours afterward, with a noticeable *heightened awareness too.*

I had felt this same heightened awareness as a 10 year old child, when I was swimming in deep water off a rock outcropping of the Mexican coast. Just at the outer edge of visibility, which was about 100 feet, were huge shadows appearing and disappearing through the murky shadows. They were whales, and they started to sing! And though I heard the song with my ears, I also felt the reverberation on my skin and throughout my entire body. I remember feeling as tiny as a mouse, and frightened – but absolutely exhilarated at the same time.

That experience has stayed as a bright light in my memory for all these years; and was the inspiration for *Private Island*, one of my instrumental albums, which also includes the song of these precious humpbacks intermingled with the music. I still have the oil painting I made for the CD cover hanging upon my wall. Bringing the picture to life by choosing the palette of colors, how the sun hit the water, etc., brought out that same feeling in my senses that I had felt over 30 years previously. When the time came I could paint and compose everything I needed from that very strong and beautiful memory just as if it was yesterday.

A strong memory is like that, and the more senses are utilized with the memory, the stronger it will be and the longer it will last. I continue to be entrained to the memory, and to whales, so much so that on whale watching excursions I can move my hand out across the horizon and feel where they are dancing below the salty depths. This entanglement actually occurs with everything we have ever been in contact with, and is a tool we can access for much good and useful information. It is also useful with the healing work, and has led to visions popping into my head of former clients when they are in crisis, which activates an intention of prayer in their behalf. Often it is not long after that I receive a phone call or email validating the emergency, and often the miraculous outcome.

Truly, we are all connected, but it helps our brain to have a strong address to link to, which brings that information out of the static on the radio dial, out of the great stream of consciousness, and into a pin-point for a specific intentional outcome.

In constantly being the scout bee that starts the dance, we can get tired, and sometimes we need to just rest and feel comfortable in our surrounding situation, and have confidence that we can periodically entrain to the vibes around us. This helps us find *a balance within the harmonic frequencies of other creation,* of which we are also part and parcel. Sometimes we just need to "hum along" again. By spending time in the wilderness, by the sea, in the desert - all these things help us to do just that. It is a subconscious need. That is why we buy mood tapes and nature fountains of ocean waves crashing, birds warbling, crickets chirping, streams babbling, wind, and other outdoor sounds. Not only because it relaxes us, and helps us to sleep and meditate, but because it blends a tranquil frequency down into very our cells. This is also why we love going to botanical gardens and zoos. It is why getting away from it all and traveling to national parks and going out on vacation is so welcome in our lives, and necessary to maintain balance.

Cell Memory, the Five Senses, and the Holographic Brain

36

While in the physical "home" body, we view our environment primarily through the five senses. Out of our body, we view it differently, as we do not have any of the physical senses to judge things by. Let's see how this works. If I give you the word "Elvis," what do you see in your mind's eye? Sideburns, dark hair, leather pants and a crooked smile? These are all impressions of the eye, a memory retained through physical ocular vision. And through the physical memory retained by the ear, when you think of Elvis are you hearing the song *"Jail House Rock?"* Your physical cells are recalling saved sensory memory as hearing and sight are being accessed. It is quite possible to have other physical memories brought up with this one word too - perhaps the memory of exactly where you were, and what you were doing, when you heard of Elvis' untimely death. Cell memory tape-records to our brain, and even our physical body.

Smells and taste also stimulate memory, and a strong cellular action can place you back in a time or thought almost immediately. Perhaps the taste of apple wine remembers a moonlit blanket and a lover's kiss; perhaps the smell of a lily remembers a date pinning the flower on your dress for prom. Perfume and cologne manufacturers know the power of scent well, and millions of dollars are spent every year to stimulate subconscious desires and memories, with a large return back. Is it any wonder most women scent their bodies to make themselves more appealing? On a subconscious level, she is planting memories within the male psyche, which will aid him to keep in mind the pleasurable time they had together, which can easily be remembered later.

I have found the body remembers even when our minds can't. Many times I've been with a client and have had my hands grow hot over a place of old trauma. I will make mention of it, and ask when or how the area got injured (sometimes I will also get a corresponding number in my mind - a year, month or age date to stimulate their memory). Sometimes they will say something like this: *"Oh yes, I remember now, I had a hunk torn out of me from a dog bite when I was eight - but that was 70 years ago!"* or *"Now I remember, that's the place where my arm was shattered 27 years ago!"* The body remembers, and stores cell memory and cellular trauma, for good or for bad, and operates like an "Akashic record" for the life of the body.

Other times, they will not remember anything for a few days, and then it will come to their memory. Often as a physical area heals, the corresponding emotional overlay heals as well. Conversely, *this is also why a physical area will not heal when the emotional psyche refuses to let it go.* This is why forgiveness and willful intent to move through old traumas and let them go is crucial to the client receiving a good physical healing.

If the client is in a good mental attitude, the cell memory records can be relieved or wiped cleaned through Divine healing. Have you wondered why the older a person gets, the more aches and pains are felt? Now you know - the body remembers. Often this is not useful for us, and we can choose to let this go, and the corresponding lightness will bring back a sense of youth that we DO want to remember!

Now, what makes this more interesting is when I am *not holding my hands over a place of injury.* Perhaps I am in first position, with hands just lightly placed upon the head of the client - and yet I still know the locations of injury on the body, and the client feels heat occurring in those areas. It has nothing to do with physically touching that particular place, though I am still getting information. According to Pribram's theory, that is because the brain speaks in the language of wave interference and analyzing frequencies; we operate like a radio on a certain band-width, we understand our world only by resonating with that portion of it. Experiments have also shown that consciousness and memory are *not localized in the brain,* but is available *everywhere* in our body - we literally are living in a holographic mind - one spot has all the information that every other spot does.

OK, let's take this one step further. An older woman comes in with unknown pain in her stomach, and she feels nauseated and has high anxiety. *I find nothing physical,* and look deeper and find a definite energy imbalance over the solar plexus and vaginal area. It does not seem linked to any prior sexual abuse, which can also show as emotional and/or physical injury in this area. As I steady my mind and open to the connection of prayer, I see an unhappy young blonde woman in her 20's who is pregnant. I describe to the client what I am seeing. *"Oh my God! That's my daughter! I think about her all the time, she is going through so much, 6 months pregnant and her husband is gone, and she doesn't work you know, I just don't know what I'm going to do..."*

What is going on here? This woman has tapped into her daughter's trauma and is experiencing pain from it, because they are entrained. When it is brought to the attention of the client of what it is and where it is from, this gives the client the ability to release from it and is encouraged to re-direct her energy to be a powerful reflector of love rather than a weak receiver of pain. This situation happens numerous times with bonded partners, and in many relationships of care; whether it is husband and wife, father and son, mother and daughter, brothers and sisters, or even just excellent friends. It also happens conversely when we can't let go of anger toward a divorced mate, unfaithful lover or cruel parent. The connection to one another *is real,* and our body knows it, and shows it, whether for good or bad. But we also have the Free Will to recognize it and use it only for positive impact on the world.

We are the Interpreter of What We See

Knowing that we are connected to one another and to every event that has ever happened in any place or time is a very useful insight for the OOB (out of body) or RV (remote viewing) practitioner. However, it can also be an overwhelming one. Our advanced mind is a sophisticated signal receiver, but we have to decode it ourselves, since we alone are the interpreter of what we see. This personal interpretation makes important differences in what kind of information we can accurately perceive, without misunderstanding or clouding perceptions because of previous trauma, lack of experience, or particular training.

For example, I know nothing about military installations, types of planes and technical equipment, or political history and espionage. I would not be a good candidate for accessing information on this - whereas someone with a background in these things will have a much more accurate hit rate. I just have nothing in my background the information can be related to. However, finding a missing person I can do very well with. Any injuries call out to me strongly; I have a natural compass in my head for direction; and I am personally familiar with many zonal areas of the United States and what grows there. Also a plus, (sorry fellahs) the built-in maternal drive is very intense to sooth and nurture children as quickly as possible. So, I would be a logical candidate for interpreting clues quickly on a missing person case, but not for any military agendas.

Developing Strong Intention, Power of SPI (Specific Prayerful Intent)

Everything we are going to do starts as a mere thought in our mind. There is no scientific way to prove thought is there; there is no mass, no speed of acceleration or measurable quality of definition that I know of. But, it is the seed where entire new cities and civilizations are germinated; the new libraries are written; the new medications are developed; and the new peace treaties are signed. It all begins with a single, intangible thought.

Now, how does a person develop a strong enough purpose to be successful at these thoughts, to bring them up into manifesting a real outcome? Initially, if you have a hard time with understanding the power of your mind, you can *jump-start* strong thought processes by *utilizing personal cell memory*. Then you can choose from any number of memories and experiences, from the past, present, or even the future (more on that later). Strong memories stimulate strong emotions. Strong emotions emit power. Power emits energy. Energy combined with SPI (specific prayerful intent) can create all things. A strong prayer life manifests much power and positive change by the connection to Supernatural outcome, as your intention touches the face of All There Is, and He responds in kind to the positive reality. When we choose to entrain our vibration to His Divine vibration, we move out of the chaos and static into pure stereo tone. It is "our will be thy will," that place of allowing Free Will to resonate and entangle within the quantum pulse. It is where everything happens, everything manifests, and miracles become common place. It is the everyday life of the mystic.

Developing strong focus is a good practice to utilize in many places in your life. It keeps you in control of your actions and emotions, and not in a state of constant re-action to your environment. For accessing cell memory, all you need to do is fully remember something wonderful in your life, utilizing all of your senses. That's all! Then bring that memory/mood/frequency to your present situation. This is actually a process of self-entraining, and you can do it whenever you like.

For example, you are stuck on the freeway in rush hour traffic, and the traffic is backed up for miles because of an accident up ahead. Everyone around you is impatient and following far too closely to one other. With a scowl on your face, you are probably (consciously or subconsciously) picking up on others non-verbal impressions of *"who cares, just get the junk out of the way and let me through, why does someone have to get creamed on my watch - I'm late!"* Now, you have a Free Will choice with this. You can continue to have a bad reaction to the actions around you and resonate to these lower vibrations, or you can entrain them to your higher one, put a smile on your face, and emanate love and positive intentions to all those around you. It will make a difference, to you and to others, and you will be creating a positive ripple effect for the ones in the accident as well.

Remember the musical instruments humming along with the piano note? It wasn't by conscious choice of the instruments, something else was happening here. With each moment, you have an opportunity to help not only yourself, but those around you, even without their knowing about it. I am aware of only very few cases where another person's core of Free Will has rejected such an offering. Most people really do want to feel good, be energetic, be worry and pain-free, and will allow themselves to resonate with that higher frequency. Most people want to feel love in their lives. Yet some do not. You can help.

Focus on a beautiful, loving memory. Totally immerse yourself in it. Maybe it is a scene from a vacation you took in the California Redwoods with your husband and children. *See* the huge trees towering up into the sky, their lush canopy shading all the tall slender ferns underneath on the mossy green forest floor. *Feel* the cool dampness on your skin, *hear* the soft murmurs of a hidden trickling creek. *Taste* the sweetness of the apple in your hand, as you gather on the quilted blanket to eat a picnic together, *smell* the ginger baked salmon. *Bring in all your senses.* Make it real! Let the joy and bliss flow through you, allowing yourself the connection with Love. You are making a specific prayerful intent (SPI). You are co-creating your world, in a positive way.

41

Don't worry that this focusing seems harder than you thought - yes, it will take some practice. When you first begin, it may be difficult to go beyond utilizing any more than *two* senses at a time. But your positive past memories can be invaluable aids for you, and everyday is an opportunity to make more of them! When you recognize an experience that you would like to remember later, clearly touch, taste, feel, hear and see everything intensely around you, intentionally committing it to memory. Always be looking for the exciting and playful, since these can be recalled quite easily. Choose experiences where your emotions are really involved. Perhaps its the memory of holding your first child; how lovely she looked, the first squeaky cries, the sweet humid smell, her soft bodily warmth in your arms, the salty taste of your own tears of joy... Whatever memories you can bring of a higher vibration into your present situation will immediately affect change in your energy and the energy of those around you. Give it a try, and you will be amazed.

You are learning to empower yourself while making a cognizant decision to benefit yourself and everything around you. You are becoming a very bright spot on the planet.

"Psi meaning comes through emotionally intense visual, auditory and kinesthetic experiences. It is a human potential we can learn to tap. We can use our intentionality as a probability perturbation instrument. We can use mental focus to alternately concentrate and relax our attention. Intent is suggested as a variable in transmission and reception in the exchange of extrasensory information, possibly within the range of ELF electromagnetic frequencies." - Sidorov, 2002

More suggestions and a few games for developing focus can be found in a later chapter, where strong intention is listed as an aid to intentional bilocation.

Meditation

There are multitudes of books on meditation, so I will be very brief here. Yes, it is necessary to know how to quiet your mind from bouncing around everywhere. It is true that the quiet mind is the canvas on which wonderful scenes can be painted, if merely given the chance. Yet one form of meditation that works for one person may not work for another, both in method, duration or consistency. Meditation is a sacred place where you can hear both the whispers of God and your higher consciousness, and you will need to experiment with what works best for you.

For me, prayer is that place I live in an undertone of Connection - it is not a place only about *asking,* but of *receiving.* Since I am always listening, I am always hearing. I hear wonderful things – even spontaneous *do it now* things, when I get the word to NOW take the next exit, NOW make a left turn…and then I witness an accident happen, and "by coincidence" I am first on the scene to aid with healing. I hear and see many things, and not all are life-and-death matters, but they are all opportunities to make changes by SPI. I hear the house plants cry out when they need watering, and when rain needs to come into the forest. Fifty miles away I see my cats chasing each other through the living room about to knock things over, and a car starting up the mountain way too fast for the sharp turns. SPI allows changes even seconds before an event, and in this place of co-creating, even shifts in time concerning the event and its ripple effects.

Therein lays the proof that one is living with full connection in the universe. When you are able to live life in this undertone, you surrender many things. You surrender worrying about tight schedules (I have found Spirit can't read clocks - or doesn't want to); what other people think (you say what you have to say, and do what you have to do); where you end up practicing your modality (such as surrounded by people in Disneyland Park), and still trust in the process wholeheartedly! It makes for incredible experiences, and a bunch of them. Life never gets boring when you have "one ear to the heavens and one to the earth."

While living in this undertone current - let's say 110 AC - I might want or need to amp up, really focus attention, and plug in to 220 AC. How will I do this? I will make a SPI (specific prayerful intent) to Father. The Big Guy and I are tight - the near-death experiences and stigmata have sealed that deal! We talk casually, like a conversation between respected and beloved friends. There are no magical words to say on my part, or any need to manipulate and approach him like a celestial Santa Claus. He is the personification of Ultimate and Unconditional Love, knows the bigger picture of everything, and I absolutely believe and trust Him. I would *never* try to use only my own power and strength for any of the modalities, healing or otherwise. It would, at best, be an awkward dance that would lead the bees off into barren fields and destruction, with no honey making back at the hive. The Connection is where the Power is, the power motivated by Unconditional Divine Love.

I have seen way too many healers and intuitives who are suffering from exhaustion, depression, and have numerous odd diseases and undiagnosable maladies. This is from using your own energy through the years, and getting other's stuff on you, which is what we were talking about when a person ends up with his own vibes being lowered to those around him, instead of visa-versa. When this depletion occurs, coming back into balance can take a long time, since new thought patterns (tape-recordings) have to be created and maintained. The old patterns are so familiar, it is easy to fall right back off again and play the old tired song once more.

This repetition of behavior is not because it is good for you, but simply because you are familiar and accustomed to it, and it takes an active choice to change the programming. So, it is a good habit to just start off the right way - and spending time in the silence will help you live in that undertone of connection at all times, and that way you never have to come back to it, *because you have never left it.*

The Celestial and Terrestrial Environments

The celestial environment is very different from the terrestrial one. With some modalities, you may be fully out, but with others, it is more beneficial to be at least part way in. We are now going to compare the differences and similarities between distant healing, which I consider a *celestial environment* (with the healer in the out-of-body state); and remote viewing, which I consider to be a *terrestrial environment,* with the viewing occurring while still very much grounded in your body. We will go further into the how and whys of both of them in later chapters, but lets just look at something interesting that was brought up by analyzing the results of my preliminary study with the Distant Healing Research Questionnaire. This information has changed my entire method of distant healing, and the protocol of how I remote view; perhaps it will also aid you. If you wish to skip ahead to read the chapter with the entire questionnaire, that is your option. But we are going to also cover a few questions from the study here with reference to the differences of Distant Healing (DH) and Remote Viewing (RV).

Remote View for Medical Intuition and Spiritual Communication - NOT HEALING

(63). <u>If you were given Medical Intuitive/*PHYSICAL HEALTH* notes by the healer after the DH treatment, were they accurate?</u> Yes! Completely accurate (65%) Most was accurate (9%) Two or more was accurate (7%) I do not know yet. I have yet to be checked by a medical professional (6%) Only one detail of the medical information was accurate (5%) I told the healer everything before hand. Nothing was new (4%) None of the medical information was accurate (3%) N/A (1%) Other (0%)

(64). <u>If you were given Medical Intuitive/*EMOTIONAL HEALTH* notes by the healer after the DH treatment, were they accurate?</u> Yes! Completely accurate! (63%) Most was accurate (11%) Two or more was accurate (8%) Only one detail of the emotional information was accurate (7%) I told the healer everything before hand. Nothing was new (5%) None of the emotional information was accurate (4%) I do not know yet. I have yet to be checked by a mental health professional (2%)

From these two questions, we see that the accuracy level of the intuitive notes for emotional and physical health was rated very high by the client.

Often during remote viewing for medical intuition I can see the layout of the rooms, the gray cat jump on the bed, the children sleeping in their beds down the hall, the color of the client's hair, what they were wearing, and clear medical details. But, further study on the questionnaire showed that while the

45

client was indeed happy with all this information, *actual physical healing was much less.* So, I came to an important conclusion:

Item #A - On the healing nights that I "saw" more things, *less physical healing occurred.*

The distant healing was more like a *remote viewing event* which gave good *medical intuitive* information and *emotional intuitive* information, rather than becoming a physical healing event. This could not easily be seen by the questionnaire statistics being taken as a whole - but within the body of each answer and outcome. Also, the remote viewing aspect seemed more conducive to #65 - which included the healer receiving information for the client from persons who had died, or other beneficial entities (such as saints and Angels) and visions.

(65). If you were given ADDITIONAL INTUITIVE notes by the healer after the DH treatment, did they include: *(listed by category, clients were asked to mark all that applied. This question has a "no entry" percentage of (12%).* Words, image or contact from: someone who had died (42%) Visions of items, places, homes (33%) Saints or religious figures (21%) from God (21%) pets who had died (12%) someone still alive (5%) Other (2%)

This information was much more prominent with remote viewing than with true distant healing, which was conducive to communication by me with the other side, but was more difficult to bring back from my conscious memory in good detail. Large conversations accurately written from DH celestial memory were rarely able to be written down, whereas the RV terrestrial environment allowed physical writing or speaking at the actual time of connection, since I had full use of my physical mouth to make audible comment to my secretary, who then typed it down.

Distant Healing Best for Physical Work, Manifestations - NOT INFORMATION

(52). Did you wake up during the DH? YES (60%) NO (40%) If so, please continue: *(listed by category, clients were asked to mark all that applied.)* I felt a tingling sensation (72%) I felt a warm sensation (70%) I felt I was not alone (63%) I was not aware of any unusual feeling when I woke up (26%) Saw an image of the healer in the room (24%) Saw a mist, apparition, or image in the room (17%) saw an image of Christ, Angels, or other religious figure in the room (8%) Did any of these images appear as solid (NO 88%) YES (12%) hear any unusual sounds (12%) smell any unusual odors (10%) Other: (14%) *NOTE: "Other" included light in the room; vibration of the bed, hands or face working over the body; seeing colors; hot sensations; animals acting strangely and waking the client up; and details of "unusual sounds" or "smells" (i.e. roses, voice calling name) etc.*

Item #B - On the nights that I simply connected for healing, more physical healing, manifestations and apparitions occurred.

The best healings occur when I simply become free of my body and connect in the Oneness, and see the person glow as the unity occurs. I can feel more Energy moving through me, and through them, and their whole body grows in brilliance. And these people experience extraordinary physical healing, and yet I may only have one or two intuitive things to relate when I get back. These are also often the prime occasions when a mist or image, apparition or physical body appears in the room. This stage also correlates with more people being awakened by vibrations or heat occurring. Sometimes this also creates an opportunity for bilocation.

To receive an excellent response for distant healing or for remote viewing, the connection needs to be strong between the client and the healer. Now let's look at how to establish that, so the very best possible outcome is available for every person that you desire to help, even without having ever met the person before in real life. This also applies to creating an excellent connection between you and the client while together in the same room, in a hands-on situation.

Recognizing the Defining Moment –
Expecting the Miracle through Client/Healer Resonance

"I do not ask how the wounded one feels, I, myself, become the wounded one." – Walt Whitman in *Leaves of Grass.*

"The flesh is the test of the spirit...love one another...welcome to the world of healers..." - Christ's words at my lightning strike - Tiffany Snow.

A personal defining moment often acts as a catalyst for a client's ability to receive healing, and for a healer to give it. Often the healer needs to have personally recognized a defining moment (often through a "wounding") and the suspension of belief that allows immediate healing beyond the mind-set of current reality. The client must also be encouraged to recognize such a suspension, to participate in activating their healing beyond common conventional ideologies or statistics.

(1). There are two ways of receiving information - through that which we choose to *believe* and through *experience.*

Empirical experience may force a change in long-held convictions, along with a reorganization of priorities in one's life. Sickness, a near-death experience, loss of a loved one, relationship and financial devastations, and numerous other traumas are opportunities which can stimulate new states of awareness beyond previous beliefs. Now, instead of persons going along with the crowd, they are making new decisions for themselves, trusting their newly-awakened inner knowledge. A shifting of awareness occurs. New priorities are set: spending more time with loved ones tops the list; job advancement and material excesses are pushed to the bottom of it.

(2). A person has only two choices at a defining moment, to move toward *positive* change, or to succumb to the *negative.*

No outside influence has a final say over personal Free Will, it is the individual choice of the one involved. Intuitively, every person knows that no one, and nothing, can manipulate another person's mind unless he allows it. From a defining moment onward - which may start with a diagnosis of an illness - some will choose to stay within a victim mentality, and no amount of conventional or integrative therapy will facilitate a healing with them. They

48

have told themselves there is no hope. No medicine, technology or caregiver can heal them, because they do not see it as possible. Outwardly they may profess desire for the treatment; but it is something being done to them. Inwardly, there is no personal responsibility to accept a positive outcome. They have given up, they feel *hopeless.*

It is important for us, as caregivers, to offer ourselves as joint companions in the process of healing, to encourage the client's personal responsibility for holistic outcomes. When this happens, tremendous advances can occur; emotionally, spiritually and physically.

Those who choose a positive outcome from their defining moment will live successful and meaningful lives, whether the physical body fully heals or not. These are the ones whose eyes smile with gratitude for every breathing moment; and who's every word is brimming with exuberance and vitality. They are the ones eager to care and to share love and encouragement with others - no matter what their own situation may be. These are the people who see the ended relationship as a new beginning, as an opportunity to know themselves more intimately, and to learn that being alone and being lonely are two different things. These are the ones who see surviving the car accident as a miracle, instead of being angry at God for the crash in the first place. These are the ones who spend all their time creating and sharing works of art to brighten the world - as they learn how to hold a paintbrush between the teeth of their quadriplegic body. It is the mind-shift that occurs when the experiencer of negative circumstances firmly states: "I don't BELIEVE I will get well – I KNOW I will!"

These are the ones who *become stronger in the broken places*, and allow themselves to become rebuilt into the true potential they were created to be, with a burning desire to fulfill their life purpose. This passion aids a return to health to fulfill that need. This is where the healer steps in, and a partnership can unfold, creating a place of quantum resonance and entrainment.

From the healer's side, when the defining moment appears, she firmly states: "I don't BELIEVE healing works – I KNOW healing works." Together in combination, the healer and client create a common ground where fertile seed

49

is sown for receiving healing. Then both expectantly wait together as the winter storm passes of ill health, the rain stops, the sun comes out, and Gracious spring offers His bounty of wholeness and health. This is where all true healing can begin.

Sometimes, before we enjoy spring, we have to go through a thunderstorm. This is where *my* ultimate defining moment came from. And what I needed to jolt me back into remembrance of who I am, who He is, and who you are too: my lightning strike near-death experience.

CHAPTER 4

My Near-Death Experience(s)
And Other Initiations of Shifting into Higher Awareness

In all parts of the world, in tribal ritual or fundamental tradition in all cultures and in all periods of time, a process of initiation often foreshadowed a shift into higher states of awareness. In the ancient past, first-hand experience was the true course to supernatural wisdom, rather than relearned and passed-down information as it is commonly received today. Vision quests, dreams, unusual baptisms, fasts, isolation, self-denial and even self-mutilation were all individually perceived as touchstones to reveal personal truth and life purpose. Today in some indigenous cultures and cloistered monasteries, forms of these still continue for spiritual development. It is interesting to recognize that healing and supernatural abilities were more widely accepted, and often prized, by those communities that regarded empirical experience highly. The awakened person was considered a touchstone to the mind of Spirit.

Also prevalent in most cultures is the "lightning shaman," the stories of the one chosen by the bright electrical finger of God to heal, prophecy and lead the people along their journey. In those cultures, including Native American, I am considered one of these, chosen by Grandfather Lightning and the Great Spirit himself. I am happy to wear this title, but words do not make an intuitive or healer; connection with The Big Guy does, and we all have that Connection, and can choose to access it at any time, if we are only aware of it and wish to.

Many people throughout history have come become aware of their Supernatural connection in unusual ways. This has even included the ancient custom of exposing oneself to various substances. Hallucinogens and other ways of experiencing altered states of consciousness have been used to bring on a near-death or death-like experience. But instead of being in a "death-like" state, for many this has been a death experience, with no coming back. I will take Divine Intervention anytime over self-imposed ordeals!

Since the altered state or "coming back from the dead" has always been considered a highly prized gift, the one who survived the ordeal was thought to be newly imbued with mystical gifts. Often they were right, but sometimes the newly gifted now had brain damage or other physical impediments. Please also remember that a defining moment is not even necessary if you can see the reality of the Divine Flame and the Connection you already have with Him as a spark from that Flame.

Today there are also many tales of going beyond and coming back with special abilities and gifts, which often include healing and psychic abilities. The International Association of Near-Death Studies, Inc. www.IANDS.org is the greatest repository of near-death and death-like experiences in the world today. There are other good internet sites as well, such as www.near-death.org. My stories are only some of those listed, but hundreds are those who have literally gone to the Light and come back to tell about it. And all these experiences are accompanied by a loss of fear of death, and dramatic life changes in the lives of the individuals. Again, this is just one aspect of awakening, but one that I am most familiar with.

A bit of research will also glean many stories of Eastern adepts and Western Christian mystics attaining enlightenment. These experiences go by many names, including "opening the minds eye," "awakening to your true nature," "Shakti rising," "awakening Kundalini," etc. Often it is a direct, raw, genuine and authentic experience that words can't embrace, a moment of visitation with the All There Is. This experience can occur as a violent sudden episode that stimulates the spirit and flesh to divide, and the spirit to attain Oneness while the body goes lifeless, rigid and cold to the touch. There is often no discernable breath or circulation. I have also been drafted into one of these experiences, which is sometimes called *rapture.*

In this chapter I will share both stories of my personal initiation into advanced spiritual awareness by these methods, and also the unusual and spontaneous event of stigmata. No matter how a true experience is received, the occurrence of unity feels timeless, but the concept of enlightenment turns a timeless moment into an *all the time* fixed identity that continues beyond minutes, hours or days. It becomes a quantum *indent* of entrainment that is a

52

touch-stone for the entire life of a person. These unusual experiences become more real than reality itself, and are remembered as if they occurred only yesterday.

Could it be in our modern world, where most of our information comes second-hand, that the increasing illness, diseases, and stress-induced traumas are becoming substitute initiations to higher awareness? Are they becoming our new rites of passage? By coming to a defining moment by conquering cancer through prayer, shifting excessive alcohol consumption through acupuncture, and defeating migraines through visualization and meditation, are we creating new touch-stones to self and God-awareness?

Truly, today's new pioneers are the ones who are wresting control back of their health from the so-called "absolute" powers of conventional medicine, chemical dependent psychiatry, and fear-based religions. *It is not always effortless, but we know that great change never is.* But, it is well worth the endeavor, and this is easily reflected in the whole physical, emotional and spiritual body coming back into the full potential it was originally created to be.

With a successful foundation built, both the client and the healer's perceptions are shifted past the statistical odds of disease and wording of fear-based terminology. This places beating the odds back into the control of the Great Observer, of which we ourselves are also His hands, eyes and ears. Jointly we define a new outcome. This shift is never easy - for it is a process of "birthing spirit." The period of initiation is very similar to a woman giving birth - with cries of pain and inability to run from her contractions, she must focus, and push past her fears. And even though we recognize it is difficult, that nothing is truly *wrong,* we still have to step up to the plate and deliver. In this, she is enveloped in a great adventure which connects her to every mother since the beginning of time. As she relaxes in to it and allows the waves of birth to overtake her in full trust and surrender, it is at that point of full vulnerability and giving that heaven touches earth, and birth occurs. The mystical traveler, like the new mother, finds out that once the beautiful new state of being is here, what joy and wonder there is, and the difficulty in achieving it diminishes into the background.

53

God, Lightning and Healing Hands - My First Near-Death Experience

"Stars!" I shouted through the thunder. The appaloosa was pacing behind the chain link fence where we kept the farm implements. "Stars! You are always the one getting into trouble! Here you are, in the middle of a storm trying to find fresh grass!" I let the chain down off the shed with one hand, and I steadied myself against a wooden structure pole with the other. The horse bolted up the pasture, as the finger of God bolted down. Standing in the pouring rain with my arms outstretched, I was struck and killed by a bolt of lightning.

There was immediate excruciating, overwhelming pain - a fitful, spasmed rendition of the famous John Travolta "Saturday Night Fever" dance, and then I felt *no pain at all.* My eyesight narrowed as my body slowly slid down onto the wet earth; and all went black... This is the day I died - my true defining moment, and the day I was brought into the world of healing miracles. It also continues to be one of the best days of my life.

The next thing I knew, I found myself standing on nothing, way up in the universe, and there were distant colorful planets all around me. I could see misty pinpoints of stars through my raised right arm, and when I moved my arm back and forth it made the stars look wiggly, like a reflection on water. I felt dizzy. I had a sense of being able to see not only in front of me, but all around me at the same time. Floating just a few feet from me, I saw a man with a spirit body like mine (no wings) and he was short, had a bit of a pot-belly, and had slanted eyes. He spoke to me with a voice that I heard inside my head (telepathy), saying: "Don't be afraid, it's OK."

On the other side of me was another spirit person. He was much taller and had chiseled facial features, this one nodded approvingly at me. All the while, we were moving with great speed toward a great ellipsed ball of swirling Light; a huge orb brilliantly white in the middle and yellowish on the outside edges, like an opposite colored egg. The closer we got to it, the more I felt overwhelming Love; it seemed so warm and comforting, it encompassed my very being...like the security of a favorite grandfather's arms wrapped around

54

a child as she crawls up onto his lap.

We stopped. The bright light was still far from me. I wanted to go on - I felt like a magnet, irresistibly drawn. The desire to blend had grown stronger the closer we got. I knew it was the very Presence himself. There was an awareness that I was looking into the cosmic heart of the Great Observer of the universe. I was overwhelmed with gratitude and love.

Why had we stopped? As I stood there confused, yearning toward the Heaven beyond my reach, a glowing luminosity appeared in front of me. A spiral of golden and white sparkles formed a very tall and brilliant Angelic human form. "What have you learned?" a gentle voice asked, in a nondiscriminatory and non-accusing way. The voice was so soft and tender, yet the presence of Divine Authority was there. In my heart I had a knowing that this was the Son of God, Jesus Christ himself.

Dumbfounded, I gazed upon this figure. My mind was full of questions, which were amazingly followed by immediate answers. As I was thinking the question, the answer was there. The fear and nerve-frenzied electrical dance of the lightning strike had long since vanished, replaced by an all-encompassing sense of tranquility, peace and calm. Being from a very strict and fundamental religion, I had been taught that healing and supernatural events do not occur in modern times (and that NDEs were the result of an oxygen deprived brain); so I was in the midst of something *I had never even believed in before!*

All of a sudden, life events unfolded before my very eyes. Key moments where I had shown anger, where I had shown love, and where I had missed opportunities, appeared like a movie. I could not only see the other people from my life, but also feel their emotions. Where I had shown anger, I felt the anger and despair felt by the other person; and how it rippled on through to others because of my actions. I had never before faced the full repercussions of my choices and felt such deep sadness. Conversely, when I showed love and kindness to people, I felt the full effects of that too. The power of love rippled out from person to person, as a warm pulse triggering cause and effect in all things wonderful and blessed. I had never before experienced such joy! But the biggest revelation, sadness and incentive, came from all the missed

55

opportunities I had let go by, without doing anything at all.

Then the Christ presence said, *"The flesh is the test of the spirit...Love one another."* *"Welcome to the world of healers..."* I was told. I wanted to join myself with the Essence beyond, like a raindrop falling into the sea. But I wasn't allowed to go any farther. *"Why can't I be with you now Father? Please, Abba, Please..!"* I strained my sense of hearing and heard Angelic voices singing from the direction of the White Light. Then, a voice resonated within my body, like notes reverberating through a grand piano, and instead of hearing the words, I *became* the words in every sense of my being.

"Heal my children...Help them remember who they are..."

My whole being surrendered and I humbly offered myself for the work to be done. Instantly, I felt a child-like sense of wonderment as a flood of bliss overpowered me, and a tingling sensation filled me to my very toes, like warm liquid honey flowing through my body, starting at the top of my head on down. What was happening to me?

I was receiving an awakening, an anointing to become the true potential I was originally created to be; a soul in full connection with God and all other things. It is what we are *all* created to be.

My near-death experience encompasses many exciting details not shared here; including many other details about what is it like on the other side. But since it is published fully in my first two books and all other the Internet (it is considered one of the best), I won't repeat it here. But I wanted to highlight one other detail - I was given the choice to stay, or to come back to earth. Yet, standing before the spiraling aurora borealis of Unconditional Love, I was extremely aware of the need to make a better life review, a "better movie," and to fully accomplish the mission given to me. I also saw the need for personal change; there was unfinished business and I needed to go back and *do it right.*

What Love Is

Also please note that none of what occurred was critical judgment from God, *but only I judged myself* at the life review. Father only looks at the facets of love we have been polishing, not anything else. Even though I knew I needed to come back, nevertheless at first I begged to stay. Nowhere on earth had I experienced such acceptance, and felt the Oneness and connection between all things. And from this empirical experience, my values, philosophy and life's work would never again be the same.

From this, I learned how to love deeply (give) and to be deeply loved (receive). It is soul envelopment past the blending of bodies and minds into a Oneness that air itself cannot fit between, between the molecule and the quantum vibration of the quark, this is how I know love. It is the love that compels me and all things, and it manifests awesome power. The height and depth of this passion is beyond restraint or doubt or fear, and it whirls me as easily as a feather in a breezy canyon. And in this blending with God is a vulnerability to a point of giving up any personal identity, yet I am not lost, I simply become greater than anything I have ever been before, since I am part of all things of God. For in the true essence of Love, there is no word comprehension or safety-net, for it is a binding of energy that is felt expanding even through time, space and dimensions. This full encompassing of Love is the full essence of where Spirit lives inside me and all things, and there is no separation between anything, except by Free Will choice to be separate if one desires it.

This is how deeply I know Love, where the storms lessen and the darkness flees because of movement of heart. It is where the miracle healings begin, and the Holy Spirit reaches out His hand to crumple the knees of the blessed onto the floor. It is where the nails of the Christ live, the pouring out and rebuilding from darkness into light. And it cannot be metered or measured out, for it is fullness itself, and I feel it all, here in my heart, in my soul, in the marrow of my bones, because I love deeply, and deeply I know Love. And so can you, it is all there for you, right now and every day from now on. You are part and parcel of this Love too.

Now from that moment of Free Will surrender in my near-death experience onward, I get to be there when The Big Guy goes to work with the healings,

57

and I make Connection and then get myself out of the way. I am always booked several weeks ahead at the Institute, due to word of mouth and constant media attention. People fly in from all over the world, and most of them receive what they came for. From this first NDE, I regained purpose to my life, and became strong in all the broken places. And healing occurs for me and within my own body every time I give a healing, with all the benefits of excellent health, youth and vitality that comes with that. I also get to see the ripple effect of spontaneous and immediate healings as daily occurrences in people's lives, which gives me true joy. I have the best job in the world! And all it took was *recognizing* a defining moment, and saying *"yes, here I am,"* to awaken me to who I already am, in the fullness of Love.

Looking behind the veil with my first near-death experience gave me a glimpse of the possibilities of unlimited realities, beyond any constrictions or doubt. I know in my heart now that everything is possible, and I can make a conscious decision every day to be part of the power of Love which makes it so. I have seen the face of God, *and I am awake.* I remember who I am - who you are too - and we are the same in the Oneness. And our life journey gives us plenty of opportunities for opening further to that awareness, and to experience all facets of that Love, everyday.

The Chaotic Weave of the "Wounded Healer"

As we have seen, there are many opportunities to awaken to our defining moment. It is about asking the big questions that we receive the answers that changes our concept of death, time, and what really matters. We begin to form a bigger picture, one that makes sense.

It's like this: Let's say a friend gives you a large wall hanging, tells you to keep it because it is worth a lot, and will only appreciate in value. You take it home and hang it on your wall. You just can't see what all the fuss is about - it is chaotically woven with an ugly mismatch of threads, with knots and loose threads hanging out here and there. One day you notice some brown paper hanging down from one corner, where the backing is torn. You turn the wall hanging over, see something unusual, so curiosity gets the better of you, and you tear the entire backing off. There in front of you is an exquisite woven tapestry! A landscape masterpiece of fine craftsmanship, so beautiful and exquisite, that your heart places it far above any monetary value. Then you smile to yourself, because now you understand that every piece of thread and chaotic color, every knot, is exactly where it should be. *You just weren't aware of it at the time!* Such it is with our own lives. We are the weavers of yarn, each working on a different place, at a different time, on a different scenic tapestry, in our own individual journey. Often enough, we see the knotty problems in our lives and in other's experiences and relationships, *missing the pattern behind these completely* - until we see the weave of the bigger picture.

Those who would take the path of healing often hear the term "wounded healer." This is also the case in my life, where the early tapestry definitely had a chaotic plait. Looking back on it, I see that many of these challenges wove some very intricate patterns into the warp and weft of my being. In my childhood, I had intuitive abilities, but they were quickly shut down. Insecurity, depression and abandonment issues surfaced as my parents traveled extensively. I started asking "Why?" and the big questions about God and the purpose of life at a very young age. It was hard to find the answers. By the time I was thirteen years old, I had run away, been raped, used drugs, lived with strangers in various parts of the country, and had gone to many different schools. By sixteen, I was living on my own, working two jobs, writing for the local paper, studying various religions and finishing high school. At 17, I went into a coma from a bacterial fever, lost my photographic memory and my fingernails, and almost died. One month after turning 18, I married a minister in my church and had four children in six years.

I accepted the beliefs of a very strict fundamentalist religion, whose difficult traditions of pleasing God and men felt familiar to me. I became one of their ministers in 1979, and entered the preaching and teaching work. I strictly raised the children by church standards for nine years of marriage, until the day came when the physical abuse was just too much to take anymore. I moved with the children into a women's shelter with a ruptured disk in my neck, which left me in a neck brace and on welfare for over a year. In this church, divorce was out of the question; so I was quickly ostracized from everyone I knew. But I still held to most of the strict and judgmental tenets of the church, and true to form of guilt-induced parishioners and abused women, I begged to be let back in. It was a time of growth, through part of an endless repetition of bad experiences which begged for attention - but *none* of these became a defining moment in my birthing of spirit.

In my ministry, I had been taught that NDEs were nonsense spat out by a dying brain, and that all supernatural or miraculous events had ceased at the death of Christ. Anything beyond that was a deception and a lie to mislead the naïve. I had never even read of such experiences, since they were considered banned material. In my thorough religious education, I had become quite persuasive in theological discussions, and made certain that everything was by "the Book." Of course, that meant only *my* religion's view of the Book. My path was learned knowledge. No one could logically convince me of anything else, yet somehow all this second-hand knowledge created a void and frustration within me that reason couldn't justify. Also, my life continued to escalate my challenges, putting stones in the road, then boulders across my path, and then landslides, so that no trail was even visible. Prayer always seemed to change the situation, but only momentarily, since I would gravitate back to my own victim patterns. I viewed all my intuitive gifts as evil - weakness and hateful things buried in my own soul, since I had been convinced they were tools *against* God, not *from* him.

As the years went by, I became a proficient musician and songwriter and the tie to the church weakened. I moved around the country and had a measure of success, producing three albums in the instrumental and county music field. I did get divorced, and married again, until my new spouse's infidelity brought another divorce a few years later. I continued to raise all four children on my own, and took a variety of jobs to ease the ups and downs of a struggling singer/songwriter. After several more years I came off the road, and married once again. Less than two years into my new marriage, my husband told me of his current 17 year affair with a married woman and to "just deal with it." I was crushed and heartbroken.

Here again, I found myself at another point of trauma and brokenness. I kept asking the common questions that create a "cause and effect" of blame, guilt, unforgiveness, fear and stagnation. Such questions were: *"why do people*

60

keep hurting me?" "why had God abandoned me?" "What had I done wrong to deserve this?" The cycle needed to be broken, but I couldn't see a way out. I thought maybe I *would* just deal with it and live in a loveless marriage. The children were teenagers now, and we lived comfortably on a horse ranch, with a pool, the finest automobiles, and all the material trappings of supposedly financial stability. I was so tired of starting over, and there truly seemed no real purpose to my life. I felt broken beyond compare, and there was nothing left for me. I began to have stomach aches, anxiety attacks, headaches, and to drink too much wine. I thought I would just resign myself to ignoring the problems around me, and decided it would be hopeless to try to change it, or to pray about it. Things would just get bad again, anyway.

I was at the lowest point I had ever been; I had dug my hole of victimization so deep, that I couldn't even see a glimmer of light. So, I sat on the fence of immobilization. Science has long acknowledged the relationship between emotional and physical health, and I'm certain I would have destroyed myself one way or another if lightning hadn't killed me first. Or perhaps I would have *subconsciously* invited illness into my body - which would have been an easier out than *consciously* making a decision for change. People do this all the time, that way they can be the victims of their own body, without taking any conscious responsibility for it.

Enlightenment had to occur the only way I could accept it. The Big Guy had to get my attention, since I was too stubborn to understand or accept it any other way, since I was so thoroughly entangled in the lower frequencies around me. I had to have an undeniable mystical experience, a clear and recognizable defining moment. So, that is what I got, at the end of a brilliant flash of light that can reach over five miles in length, raise the temperature of the air as much as 50,000 degrees Fahrenheit, and contain up to a hundred million electrical volts! *(NOAA's National Weather Service)*

Today, I see my entire life as a classroom in preparation for this incredible healing journey. Many struggles and blessings came across my path, each carrying their own specific burden and lessons. Some of these trappings, most of which were victim-based and religious in nature, I have stumbled on - but by tripping I've learned to lift my feet. Looking back, I realize that all the times of brokenness were simply excellent opportunities for me to choose *love* over bitterness, *love* over fear, *love* over unforgiveness. Being slow to accept these earlier invitations to awakening, I had to take the shaman's journey, the medicine man's initiation. I had to die to really start living, and it had to be Divinely induced. Hence, the lightning strike became my defining moment, and though each person's lightning comes in different ways, this was mine on my journey toward initiation into awareness.

Becoming True Potential - Moving Past Static into Pure Stereo Tone

I have further shared my life story to emphasize an important point: an initiation into higher states does *not* mean we came from living a life of perfection, or that we "earned" it in some way. Rather, it means we can accept who we are, and everyone else too, precisely *because* of our frailties and imperfections. Then each of us can be a miracle worker in our own lives and in the lives of others, in whatever form that takes. When I use the word *"miracle,"* I am referring to a *supernatural intervention beyond common recognized reality*. Miracles are a blessed intention of Divine Energy, which manifests through people who recognize the cosmic cause and effect of Love. Yes, it may (and often is) physical healing, but it is intervention in other aspects of our lives too. And I have learned it's not about *earning* love it's about *spending* it and *giving it away.*

In my own case, my highest specialization is hands-on and distant healing; I truly am in the business of miracles. But that same place of specific prayerful intent (SPI) and connection is also where I have also helped find missing children, solved murder cases, gathered information by psychic archeology (touching things and the soil), helped the FBI with 9-11, see and communicate with ghosts and spirits, conduct deliverances and exorcisms, and find my missing car keys!

The abilities available to each of us might be compared to owning a radio. Most people live in a fog of white noise, and are unaware of the stereo tones just outside of the static. By accepting quiet stillness, and *desiring to hear the whispers of the One God*, we can intentionally move through the static and tune into channels of our own choosing. Some people become comfortable with only one station; such as being tuned in to healing vibrations. However, just as there are classical, jazz, pop and many other channels to choose from, we can willfully focus on distant healing, then further to remote viewing for medical conditions, or any variety of other things. It is all about how we choose to turn the dial. *There are no limits!*

At first we may be afraid to move out toward the other channels, since every time we begin to shift out of our comfort zone, we initially hit static, much of which we actually cause by ourselves. And, as always, the naysayers are there, ready to tell us "there be dragons that live at the end of the world", and "your journey will land you in a void off the edge of the map." To them, there is no music, since they can't hear it for themselves. Their second-hand knowledge and their choices of belief say it can't be so. But all the wonderful melodies and harmonies are there; and it all comes from the same source, the high frequencies of the Great Radio Tower. All we have to do is *shift our perception of connection* to tune into the right broadcasting system, while having trust and faith in the final outcome as being real and complete.

"Now faith is being sure of what we hope for, and certain of what we do not see." (Heb. 11:1).

Fear is the opposite of love, and faith's job is to replace fear and guide us out through the chaos of white noise into the desired rich stereo tone. It helps us to trust enough to step upon the path before we even know the final destination. So, we see the *healer* needs *trust,* but is *faith* really a necessary ingredient for a client to have, in order to be healed? Over and over again, I have to say that faith implies ability and humility in receiving, letting go of unworthiness issues, and moving past fear and into love and hope. And I have seen that when there is no faith, *the healer can step in and utilize her own* for the miracles to happen in the client's stead, if the client is at least open to the possibility of positive change occurring.

In my own journey, though my initiation of my first spiritual awareness came with a "zap," even then I was left with an opportunity to cling to old beliefs, or embrace empirical wisdom. In my choice, I have come to the conclusion that a person does not need to have a NDE to activate or recognize their potential, and that we are *all* created with the opportunity of natural gifts, and can tap into the Great Supernatural ones as well.

Consumed into All There Is - My Second Near-Death Experience

Since the first awakening over seven years ago, I have had an irresistible desire to go back, a deep homesickness that has followed me around where ever I go. Uncounted times I would try to return, by out-of-body or astral travel, straining be in the Presence once more, but never quite able to do so. Then, almost six years after my first visit, my prayers were heard, and I was called back, induced by one of the most profound experiences anyone could ever hope to have, by a method I was not even aware existed.

Since then, I have found similar accounts of this experience from all parts of the world. God is like that, never showing favoritism and allowing His embrace to be felt wherever He chooses. This time He chose to bring me home again through what some might term "rapture," and I will be forever grateful.

In preparation for this kind of further enlightenment, there were many things that I had to move through, which I only fully recognized after the fact. Since detailed insights on the process of rapture are not well known (I found very little in my research) I will share these personal journal notes with you. It is always important to share what we have learned with one another, it helps all of us to advance and glow. But, I do not expect that the process is the same for everyone - yours will probably be much different from mine, as each of us is unique in what is required for us to open up and take the next big stride. In retrospect, the steps that were given to me were part of an unfolding and unburdening of physical, emotional and spiritual blockages and further alignment of my will into His will. I have listed the steps and experience below.

The Preparation and Subtle Shifts for Further Thinning of the Veil

(1). <u>Dec. 2004</u> On Sabbatical for five weeks. I usually fast for much of my

64

sabbatical time, and was planning to do so for 30 days, or a little over four weeks. But at only a little over 2 weeks into the fast, The Voice resounded through of me – *"eat, build an altar inside your home and celebrate Communion every night."* When Father said to stop fasting I initially argued with Him, since I had found it "thins the veil" and the plans had been given to write a new book. Previously I was celebrating the Eucharist, or Communion, once a week. Nevertheless, I obeyed. I covered a nightstand with a purple cloth, placed a crucifix, candles, incense, Holy water, frankincense and the consecrated host and wine upon it, along with some personal sacred items. I placed a large pillow for kneeling on the floor in front of it.

The first night a most glorious event happened, which had only previously occurred at my near-death experience. While I was down on my knees finishing my prayers, I heard something just on the outside of my hearing. Straining my ears, the sound became louder and louder, until I physically heard a heavenly choir of Angels singing - and unlike last time, I could understand the words! I was experiencing what I had heard nearly 6 years before at my first NDE - the singing of Angels praising God! Tears came to my eyes, it was so beautiful, and it was a welcome reminder of one of the most beautiful experiences of my life, knowing Father surrounds Himself with song. I knelt there and cried as my heart overwhelmed with joy. It seemed like this particular fasting/purification time and then following His words closely, opened a new level of opportunity for me, since immediately after this is when I also experienced my first bilocation.

The following italicized info is a possible summary of my lessons learned.

Breaking with personal tradition, incorporating new rituals. Divine validation of progress. Obedience has its rewards.

(2). An energy shift occurred in the healing work, whereas before the Holy Spirit seemed mostly channeled *through* the body. Now it seems to go around, over and through my body *all at the same time,* and I am like a log in the river current of Spirit, and I control the amount and direction of flow. Less tenderness now on top of head after healing, body loses appetite, increase of water intake, rapid weight loss begins. Less need to "insulate the electrical cord," as body fat had increased after lightning strike/healing initiation. Spirit energy is shifting in much wider circle around me. More electrical problems increase in a wider radius around me including lights now surging in lobby and front office, including video, TV and computers shutting off. I cannot go anywhere near credit card machine or computers once the healing day has started, and client's watches are reported to still be breaking after putting them back on more than four hours after the session. Instant healings show a definite increase in quantity, as my ability to be a wider channel increases the ability for the client to pull through what they need and will accept at the moment, without any clogging whatsoever on my part.

Surrendering shift in energy while maintaining trust in its full capacity without having to control all of it through my own body. Seeing the humor in the worsening electrical problems without getting upset; seeing the impact of how one person's shift affects a large area.

(3). For much of my intuitive and healing life, being in crowds of people felt too overwhelming to me, since I felt a personal desire to "heal them all," whether it was requested or not. This was self-imposed, but difficult to come to grips with. Now I was going to movies, arcades, and being around large groups of people, but learning to let it all flow over me, and around me, including touching, without cringing or pulling back because of excess of information from people or objects. Not judging information anymore, just seeing it as there, letting it flow through me and transforming all of it without needing to decide who it goes to. Healing and intuition on automatic now, 24/7, the intention consciously made to be a constant flowing vessel of love to all who would accept it, without any of my personal limitations about it. This helps a lot with my ease of being around live people, with their accompanying transitioned or stuck relatives and friends. I also know that many other people are able to help with this part of the work, and that I do not need to do it all.

Letting go of fear of being overwhelmed by feeling too much. Continued lessons of non-attached observation being still a place of fullness of Love and Free Will, while being an instrument of change and transformation for all who desire it. This occurs without me having to mentally choose to or not to choose, it is now continually "on," bypassing the analytic and judgmental brain. I choose to always be a light, there is no "draining" of me, since I am only a will-full touchstone for Love, and I receive as I give.

(4). <u>Friday June 17th 2005</u> Distant healing and deliverance/exorcism with named demon, one of the ancient fallen Angels, it puts up a big fight, tried to attack and come back through to our location, we prayed, and the Holy Angels won as usual. Afterward, dramatic waves of energy started, from feet to head, large surges shaking my whole body, I started going in and out of consciousness, was given prophetic information about my life, and world secrets which are to be unveiled later, which at this time is "for my eyes only." Next day exhausted, couldn't drive, body cold, stayed in sun, couldn't adjust body heat very well, spent day in meditation, prayer, sleep.

Greater challenges can bring a greater willful connection with All There Is, and ability to receive the highest of information.

(5). <u>Thursday June 23rd 2005</u> A couple flew in for consultation, she is being gifted with healing by God but has issues related to feeling "not good enough" for this work. Father's words to her had secondary implications for me, of releasing fear and even more fully embracing the gifts, of my own worthiness to receive as a child of God. Given additional information for deliverance, and new protocol in Institute: "take off your shoes, for this is Holy Ground," and "seal with a Holy Kiss (on client's hands)."

By feeling unworthy we can shut down the gifts. We are brought to one another for wisdom when we can't hear it for ourselves because our own emotions clog us up. Also, methods and personal protocol can be changed and fine-tuned at any stage of the journey.

(6). <u>Saturday June 25th, 2005</u> While visiting the Wild Animal Park in the morning, I noticed the monitor lizard and how much *calm and patience* he had, and the monitor lizard spoke inside my mind (telepathically) very plainly *"Stay a while, be like me."* Later that day, visited tame wolves, and heard what they had to say. I had an open discussion about true soul identity and relationships with a close friend. Went to a large birthday party, was again led to freely talk, mingle and touch people, and actually sought them out, without restraint or hesitation on my part.

The Enlightenment of Rapture

Later that night, tried to do another distant healing, waves of vibrations started again, from bottom to top. Couldn't make contact to God without stimulating the pain, even larger contractions and spasms than last time. Very painful, plainly heard Father calling me to come to Him, felt like I was dying. Struggling, resisting surrender, fighting. Fear of separation, anxiety about being exposed to the Unholy, the Demons, could feel and see them against an invisible barrier outside the house. I could see through the house as if it were glass. Could see four Holy Angels inside the house, and was aware of a large additional one on the roof. Realization that I could actually *see* Angels now, which was difficult and intermittent before, since before I had to raise my vibration extremely high, and they had to chose to lower theirs, for me to catch even a glimpse of them.

Hard energy contractions continue, couldn't release the fear, feels like birth, surging up over and over again. Could see myself as a raindrop falling into the ocean and disappearing, not knowing what was mine or others, I had a big fear of loss of identity. At one point, I could not see with my physical eyes at all, all was black, I was literally blind. This was most frightening as well. *"No, I'm not ready," "I'm scared,"* I was fighting against releasing, and ended up on floor, could not get past my fear, felt like I would lose myself, felt the Oneness calling, and was afraid of letting go, felt I would not know the difference between me and the table, me and the floor, me and a speck of dust.

Body contractions strengthen even more, as though pushing stage now during labor. I repeated *"no, no, no"* over and over again. It was reported by friend/secretary that three different languages were spoken at this time, which to him sounded similar to Polynesian, Italian and American Indian. Struggling was constant, and my consciousness was in and out of body many times. I held onto fear and kept clinging to body, unwilling to make the final release, though I had prayed for this for years, to see the focused presence of God again. This continued for several hours. Couldn't handle it anymore, collapsed and fell asleep. My friend left after being assured by Father that I would be alright.

Woke up later, found that normal astral travel was possible, and I went to the house where I had earlier been with the wolves, and spent some time with them and calmed them down. They felt comforted, did some healing on them as well. Did a much-needed sanctification of their owner's home, and spoke to the two ghosts that were there, and got them to move on and stop interfering, all while in the astral body.

I also found I could move physical things very easily now, so I did! The house sitter noticed the folded shirt and moved items the next day; and without me telling him, he asked me if I had been there and done these things. Later when the owner returned, a remark was made about a difference in energy, how the house felt, and the calmness of the animals. I was amazed that I could now move physical things while in spirit form, and so easily at that, by simple intention.

The next day there was still a physical glow around everything I saw, and I spent the morning giving a full third of my possessions to the poor, I felt strongly the need to simplify and clean out my physical living space. Only one thing is needed, maybe two. All day I felt as if I were suspended in a state of grace over the edge of a cliff, times of full awareness, all questions having immediate answers, while wide awake, simply by the intention of wanting to do so. I could gaze into the depths of this great chasm but was not falling into it, it was almost like being held back by someone hanging onto an invisible belt around me. *Saw glimpse of eternity, all knowledge, everything alive, and the need to care for the earth.* Physically good energy, active. I spent the day looking at the world through eyes that could see that all awareness was possible, at all times, *even while fully in the body.*

Physically, I saw the life-force easily perceptible in all things, *even inanimate objects. Finding desire to go further, to fall off the cliff, but not knowing if chance will come again, although still hoping it would wait a week or so, for a recovery time.* I could still feel my fear holding me back, and I knew that is what caused me the pain and fright of the session the night before, when God

69

was calling me to blend, and I was afraid.

Using Free Will to fight against what has been requested by Free Will in the first place can become a painful and repetitious physical and emotional problem for the spirit, and creates a struggle in letting go.

Finally Releasing the Fear, Enveloped by Love

(7). <u>Sunday June 26th 2005 Rapture Enlightenment – 2nd NDE</u>
Tried more distant healings, this stimulated the waves of energy once more. Not wanting to end up on the cold floor again, I lay down on the bed, and asked to hold the hand of my friend, who continued to pray out loud. Using scriptures, recognizing the balancing grace of the sanctification of the Christ, calling on the Angels to assist, trusting in Father God, letting go, surrendering, *"we are all His anyway,"* letting go of preconceived notions. Another two hours of struggle and pain, and fear of the unknown, fear of death, identity loss, etc., fought...*then finally released,* able to release, *"yes, yes, I will go...please, Father..."*

Bad muscle spasms, choking, gagging, couldn't breathe, pain in all stigmata points of body, as if Christ was there, His nails in my hands, feet, left shoulder extended out, under right rib/liver cut, back slashed, head gashed. Body no longer fought or struggled, complete surrender. *No pain, no holding back. Complete and utter trust. Sublime communion.* Explosively sat up, gasping, choking, stopped breathing, fell back on bed, skin became cold and the body died... (body cold and rigid for about 30 minutes, and without breath, attested to by friend).

"Our <u>pain</u> is the breaking of the shell that encloses your understanding."
- Kahlil Gibran.

My spirit went to God, where I saw all and became all. My friend ascertains that warmth started coming back into the body after half an hour, I was "out" for the whole time. *I became the raindrop that falls into the sea, and I did not lose my own identity, but became greater than I'd ever been, and found out the entire sea is only a raindrop as well.*

70

I asked to go through this learning slowly. Free Will creates ability to unplug from Love and create an empty chasm around us, and Free Will gives us the ability to plug back in again and see that separation is only an illusion by our own choice. Much further awareness than from previous day looking into the void, but seeing now there is no void; *all things are fully part of the whole, and the whole is part of all things.* We live in the holographic mind of God, the Great Observer. He lives through us, and the brighter we are, the more He experiences life through us. Light and darkness cannot dwell together, a person of light is a vessel for God to work through, Free Will causes separation or communion, depending on each human choice.

True communion is trade, He lives in us, we live in Him, He consumes us, He feels everything, and we feel Him. *Jesus was the first time any human was Light enough for Father to experience life fully through, including pain and suffering, and death.* At times He chooses to use this biggest experience of feeling human to connect with us and let us know He is here, that He knows us even in the marrow of our bones, He has felt pain and suffering too. This is true communion. It is a trade, a sharing of all we are, to Him. This realization was further emphasized later through the stigmata. - *When we finally surrender all things, we gain everything and have lost nothing but fear.*

(8). Monday June 27th, the Day After the New Awakening
Woke up from sound sleep to big sounds outside, like giant trees breaking, cracking wood, and thuds over and over again near the house, as if impact of close target practice with bombs. Both cats were in the windows, looking out, and looking back at me, scared, ran under the bed. It lasted maybe three minutes, some kind of shift in the land itself, around my house. I was exhausted, slept and went in and out of consciousness all day, and cold again even in the sunshine. Joint and muscular pain, fogginess of eyes and in hearing, and there was an aura around all things.

In such a state of surrender and compassion I did not want to kill bugs or even eat in case it causes harm or lack somewhere else. Then further Divine information and realization of transformation of energy, rebirth, all life wants to blend and absorb each other in the truest sense, all beyond fear and in love,

71

consumption is OK. Sex, eating, breathing, working, all things are made for the balance of communion, of consuming in trade, of giving all and receiving all. There is no separateness. There is no death, only a shift in energy.

All knowledge is available now, and any question I had was immediately answered, just as it was while I was in the heavens with the lightning strike experience. It is there for all of us, and I learned from Father that we were created as co-creators. Not just about having babies, but our power of intention to manifest things. But since the fall of mankind and other reasons, we are in a less-than-perfect state; not all of our intentions are good for us or others. For example, if we see a car coming toward us and it flickers through our mind that we would swerve and hit it, that is exactly what would happen! This is how I found out what our Guardian Angels do, the ones we came in with who stay with us throughout our lives – *their primary purpose is to void any manifestations that our negative intentions would make.* So, we might have a car crash, but it won't be from that flicker of intention that went through our minds. But the good intentions are allowed to fly - and when we go beyond our own energy and intentions and Connect with God's energy in our intentions, all things good are possible and manifest – *all things!*

Many other things I learned. I also found I did *not* desire to know all things, but wanted to be surprised by the unfolding of the events of the day, *not* put intention out, but to see the beauty of His Divine interaction and people's choices in their day. I felt peace and calm beyond words, and no fear. Strong desire to escalate the work, visualizing healing conventions of thousands of people, and miracles happening on an unprecedented scale. Speaking would not be about religious things, but spiritual; and not about darkness but about brightening and remembering who we are; and about great future events soon to come in the world. And all the while, great miraculous healings would occur.

CHAPTER 5

The Truth & Misconceptions about Stigmata
Divine Regeneration, Miracles and Visions

It always amazes me how the Great Invisible always gives us enough visible stuff to help us get new realities through our analytical brain. The Big Guy always underscores who and what needs to be paid attention to. I think that's a main reason why any Supernatural event occurs, because we should pay attention, and we *will* pay attention if it's unusual enough!

Stigmata are spontaneous manifestation of wounds on a person's hands, feet, forehead and side - similar to the wounds of the crucified Jesus. Those who describe stigmata categorize these experiences as Divine or mystical. History tells us that there have been many who bear the marks of the Passion of Christ on their hands, feet, side, or brow, often with corresponding and intense sufferings. These are called visible stigmata. Others only have the sufferings, without any outward marks, and these phenomena are called invisible stigmata. I now carry all five wounds – holes in my hands, feet, and a slash in my right side just below my lung. There are also marks and scratches up my entire back, and periodically I receive scratches and indentations on my head and brow. Before this happened to me, I had no idea it existed in modern times, and really only knew about St. Francis of Assisi having had it several hundred years ago.

Now *"heal my children, help them remember who they are,"* took on a whole different meaning for me. I had met Christ at the near-death experience, and had already felt close to Him before that, but in a strictly religious way. His words of love in the scriptures had always resonated deep within me in the books of Matthew and John. He spoke openly of peace, brotherly compassion, and of an interactive loving God in a time of intolerance, political darkness and religious oppression; even though His message would lead to His death. I have further learned that His human perfection and Free Will choice gave us the grace of the balance of Adam in a perfect way. He reflected the qualities of Dad in a way that no one ever had, or ever would. I respect and love Him a lot. He truly opened the door to balance out any "Karmic" stuff that we would never have been able to live enough to undo on our own. *Yes, Christ opened the door, but all God's kids of all religions and cultures are welcome to go through it.* His is the religion of Love.

It has only been since this last year (July of 2005) that the wounds have started, and they appear for three to five days at a time when they come, which has been approximately once every month. The rest of the time they are only scars. I have kept it private; known until now only to family and friends. I also have a photo album available to those who come to the Institute and wish to see it active, since most of the time only the scars are visible. I only speak about it now because Father has told me to make it known, so I do and will continue to do so. As per instructions, I have also allowed a website *www.stigmatahealing.com* where I add more information about what I learn during the visions of stigmata, and have photos there as well. We ask that people come for healings because they need to be healed, not only to see the scars. Indeed, there is no longer any question as to Who the healer is here!

I have found there needs to be some clarification of some common misconceptions about stigmata. All this is done to promote faith over fear, and help everyone recognize that God wishes to communicate fully with His children, of which *only one* communication is the gift of stigmata. He offers inspiration and connection to all those who request it, through many different ways.

Many Others Will Be Receiving Stigmata Soon

One of the reasons this information is being released, is because Father said; *"there will be more to experience me in this way than in any other time in history, since time as you know it is coming to an end."* Please note that this information about *time* is not a fearful thing, but a wonderful change of going *past time* and into *timelessness and brightness*, a shifting from dark to Light. Yes, there will be the difficulties of "birthing spirit" along the way, but as we have already seen, this is to be expected during great change. And more Supernatural Gifts of all kinds will accompany this in those who desire a deeper connection of Love by Free Will intention, including stigmata and miracle healings.

"Be imitators of God, therefore, as dearly loved children and live a life of love, just as Christ loved us and gave himself up for us as a fragrant offering and sacrifice to God." (Eph 5:1,2)

As Time nears its end, and moves into Timelessness, time as we know it is speeding up. And it is definitely true that more people are experiencing the Gifts of the Holy Spirit than ever before. Healing, the "word of knowledge," prophecy - so many things we are witnessing as Father reveals Himself even more in this time of historical change. Stigmata at its simplest form represents the moment of true sharing of the connection of Grace, a place where God fully felt the human condition, including pain, suffering and death, and transforms it into a new beginning a new creation of peace, vitality and life. It is the Divine's way of saying, *"I understand what the human condition is, I have felt it before."*

As we have seen, darkness and light, just like good and evil, cannot exist together; and as darkness moves towards light it either has to transform into light or move away from it to survive. God is Light, and Jesus was absolutely Bright – so it was the first time that God experienced the full human condition, including pain, suffering and even death, the full rawness of humanity at its bones and marrow. So one facet of stigmata is true sharing and communion - except this time, *He* consumes us as the bread and wine.

The experience of the stigmata is also graced by a high state of peace and tranquility mixed within the suffering, and comes in waves. It is worse than childbirth, but the waves allow for *catching one's breath* between regeneration times. It is the highest connection of Divine connection I have experienced while still existing in a body. This time of utmost peace between the pain is because God wants us to feel Joy and Love above all, in this reality of Divine connection with Him, in bridging heaven and earth, the visible and the invisible, man and God, and re-creation and regeneration.

Another Reason for the Pain – Regeneration and Replacement of Defective Cellular Tissue

The pain is also about a physical regeneration of the cellular tissue itself, where much of the inherent imperfections of Adam's Free Will choice and its cause-and-effect are now replaced with Free Will choice for Love, Unity and Light. Cells are created to cry out when they are being attacked and killed – they send a subconscious signal up to the brain which then reacts by sending all kinds of helpers to protect the cells. So during stigmata, as we allow ourselves to be brightened (which also helps Father to work with us better) we also need to allow the pain of regeneration to simply wash over us without reacting as if it is something wrong. It's actually all about something that is *right*.

Galatians 6.17 Paul writes, *"I carry the marks of Jesus branded on my body."*

For those who are having a hard time with this, believe me, I understand! Just like the lightning strike and everything else that has happened to me on this incredible journey, I have had to empirically experience it myself to accept it. I am the most stubborn one of all! And I still wonder every month if it is coming again, or if it was all just a dream. Then, it shows up again, and new revelations come in that continue the story right where the last one ended. All the visions are written down, I am not left alone at all during stigmata, and all the notes will be made available in future books and future conventions, when The Big Guy gives us the *"go ahead"* to release it. Much of it is able to be released now. This book is part of that, and we have started healing prayer classes and workshops as well, and are expanding our speaking and miracle healing events. So all I can do for the skeptics is nod my head in compassion and understanding, and offer a thought that might help, because I can't make you believe it if you won't. That's why healing is placed with the words.

Experiencing stigmata without cursing God or trying to escape the pain is also an opportunity for answering one of the Original Issues presented by the first Fallen Angel; namely that every man will curse God to save his own skin. *Many will not!* And neither will I.

"For those who believe, there is no explanation needed, for those who don't believe, no explanation will suffice."

<u>Monday July 18th, 2005</u> - STIGMATA BEGINS – Personal Notes
Overwhelming desire to spend quality time in evening prayer, which is unusually peaceful and deep. Have had much burning pain in my hands and feet, and other places which correspond with the wounds of Christ, since the 2nd NDE several weeks ago. Now it is manifesting above the skin. During the prayer time and offering of the host and wine, Father starts telling me many things about the future, and I start to see the wounds on the skin in my hands and feet. First looks just like a brown area, like a burn mark. I am amazed, and wonder if it is my imagination. Since the enlightenment of the rapture, these areas have felt like red-hot iron punched through me, especially when working on clients who have cancer or other difficult maladies. I wonder what is going on! I decide to wait until morning and look again. Many dreams occur as soon as my head hits the pillow.

<u>Tuesday July 19th</u>
Woke up with large blisters where the burns were. Round circular areas on top and bottom of hands also, and same in feet, with much additional pain. Looks like holes where nails went it, feels like it too. Went to work at the Institute, no one noticed under the dim light in the rooms – only my office administrator noticed. I start to feel immense pain with the healings in all the areas of the wounds, including left shoulder keeps "popping" out of joint, and my back starts to sting in areas, and my right side. Three of my teeth on my right jaw are loose; I taste the blood going down my throat all day. Evening is worse, blisters have popped, I take off old skin, circular areas turn red, are deeper, start to bleed. I fully realize what is happening, no need to guess now. I let Father know this body is His, I surrender, let my hands be His hands, I ask for full communion. Today, I didn't tell anyone but my daughter. Divine Love will guide me in what to do. The adventure continues.

<u>Wednesday July 20th</u> - STIGMATA
Morning and evenings are the worse. Night had multitude of short "dreams"

of the suffering, and me there witnessing and also living it at the same time. In the morning, The Voice says: *"show yourself to the Priest,"* and *"This will come and go, but I will be with you always."* I call Father Francis, a priest with the Old Holy Catholic Church, a friend of mine who let me do healings at his office when I first moved to California. At the time of this first stigmata, I was not Catholic. I asked if he could come to the Institute, but I didn't tell him why. He answers he can't come until the afternoon. I call him again 10 minutes later, ask again, and he comes down, I am at the altar in my office. Later he reveals that at time of the phone call he received a rush of energy and left his house without any problems, although he was often in much pain in the mornings and it was difficult to move. When he arrives, I am on the floor in front of the altar, blood oozing freely through the hands, feet and side. "Oh my God!" he said, "like St. Francis and St. Clare, who..." Then Fr. Francis tells me part of the history of stigmata, suggests I take it easy, he says it is up to me to work or not. I choose to work, doing the healings until I cannot, until the visions come too strongly, until I can't cover up the bleeding.

Fr. Francis and I have communion together, and he sprinkles me with Holy water, and gives prayer of protection. He asks questions. I keep hearing the demons ridicule me, although the Angels are powerful around me. I am more protected than the United States President; I can see everyone in the spirit world, all of them, and the beings of darkness behind the Angels, a legion of fallen Angels, those who used their Free Will to injure and rebel. But I trust and have no fear. I ignore what the shadows are saying, they can do me no harm. Instead, The Big Guy starts giving me jokes, and cartoons in my head - it swings between scenes of the visions of scourging, then funny things, such as *"look, a new way to hold a straw!"* (straw through hand) and *"here, let me get that for you, oops!"* (falls through the holes). God has a sense of humor, and it comes at a good time for Him to share, for me to continue to handle this relentless and severe labor of love and connection, as I try to relax into the brightening.

I had been shaking almost uncontrollably, but the shaking disappears by the time Fr. Francis leaves. I feel very emotional and vulnerable. I also experienced a broad range of emotions with this first stigmata, since it was so "unreal" to me and hard to wrap my head around. I felt unworthy, very confused, very loved, full of doubt, and very blessed, *all at the same time.* Fr. Francis asks my office administrator to call him later to let him know how I am doing. Much more blood now from feet and hands, top and bottom, still I work, but I explain it, people are very moved, no one offended, I keep Band-Aids on the inside palm wounds of my hands, no blood gets on anybody. Band-Aids have trouble sticking, must change them all the time. Overhead lights keep dimming, then become brighter again. CD players have trouble playing correct speed. Difficult to walk now, going barefoot, can't wear shoes, trying to stand on sides of feet, doesn't help much. Pain gets worse, feels like "drilling" is happening at the pain sites when I am doing the healings. This is true communion. He is sharing with me, the place where He felt most human, the place of connection to humankind experienced during the crucifixion. I understand. I see the visions more strongly.

I keep hearing the lashing of the whip, feeling it stronger on my back - it startles me every time now and makes me jump, they welt up. Now I am seeing visions of the Passion. I get very thirsty, can't get enough water, but I can't hold the cup, put on counter with a straw in it. Bleeding is less during midday, early afternoon, then in the evening, gets worse again. I call my folks and let them know what is going on. They do not know what the stigmata are, mom gets upset, I remember wishing I had never told them, but I thought they should know what is happening. I feel frustrated. Phone also keeps going in and out. They ask for Fr Francis's phone number, he talks to them twice, later they do research on the internet, and say they understand now, and are proud of me, that they realize it is a blessing. I feel better, did not want them to worry. They only ask Fr. Francis, *"what can we do to help?"* Fr. Francis says, *"she is handling it very well, there is nothing to do right now."*

This evening while celebrating the Eucharist, I go to reach for the host, and notice a spot of blood on it, before I even touch it. As I watch, the entire wafer turns bloody. I bend it in half, put half in my mouth, and the other half I place in front of a statue of Mary on my home altar. She is holding the infant Jesus in her arms, a hold-over from a Christmas scene that I couldn't bear to pack away. I wonder if the blood is mine or His – I am later told that there has been research which shows in some cases stigmata blood is of a different type than the person afflicted. This seems a sound case for knowing the blood type

79

of Christ. A statue of Mary on my bedroom altar and two Angel statues have a light shiny gloss to them, and some kind of fluid is coming from them. A look in the mirror shows I also have bruises all over my body, in all sizes. It looks like I have been pelted with stones. Perhaps from Christ falling down in the street? Or did they throw stones at him too? Father says *"both."* I see the vision of this as well. Whenever the visions start, it is as if I am observing it from a distance, in third person. I see the desert, I smell the arid dryness and plants. Then as stigmata progresses, I shift into being very close to Christ and observing, then I shift into being the body of Christ, and experiencing it all first-hand. After a while of this, I see visions of all kinds of other things, as if getting to that place of surrender opens a door for me to continue to all other things beyond it. And though the pain of regeneration still comes in waves, I see other visions that do not have to do with the Passion, but visions of future events, heavenly workings, and such like. It is most extraordinary, and I learn a lot.

Thursday July 21st STIGMATA WORSENS, THEN ENDS
Wake up from another night of dreams, I drive to the Institute, almost run off the road twice, can't hold steering wheel very well, and can't drive with shoes. Ask Fr. Francis to be there again for me, before I begin the day. Blood everywhere, holes much deeper, and woke up with spear gash in my right ribcage/liver area, about 7 cm long, and deep. I keep feeling it jab in, as if going to my spine, makes me want to vomit. The holes on the back side of my hands are much deeper than in my palm, though the ones in the palms feel the worst; the skin is so sensitive there. The back of my left hand is a full centimeter across, and almost perfectly round. I can see a further puncture wound in the middle of it, where it is the deepest, and now I can see gristle and white material when the blood isn't oozing. The hole on the inside of that hand is about half that size. They are not all the way through. The strength in both of my hands has greatly diminished, I cannot hold anything on my own, but have to have someone hold it up for me, such as my water cup, and use a straw to drink. I have diarrhea and cannot eat again. I have no desire to.

The right hand wound is off-round, and slightly smaller than one centimeter, but the puncture wound is deeper in the very middle of it. Again, in these places it feel like a "drilling" is happening when the healings occur. The inside is the same as the left hand, about half a centimeter across. The ones on my feet are at over a centimeter on top, and 3/4 the size on the bottom, though the bottoms are more painful than the top. The feet bleed very much. Both hands and feet are swollen around the wounds. The back is still not fully manifested although I feel and hear the whips. It has welted but not broken the skin yet. I feel hot on my forehead, and in the mirror I see splotches of red marks. These do not manifest any stronger today. The shoulder still keeps popping in and out, with much pain involved. Head hurts, and jaw. Knees feel raw, like scraped. Basically, whole body hurts.

Bright red blood, I ask Fr. Francis if it is Jesus' blood or mine, says he doesn't know. It coagulates very fast, in a minute or less. I go to wipe it off, and it looks like strings. I say I don't know what to do with all the blood on everything at home - I don't want to treat it with disrespect - how do I dispose of it? Do I burn the rags? Do I wash them? Fr. Francis says to wash them, and anything that I rinse out, to pour the water/blood out on the ground. We do communion again, and he looks at the pattern of the blood on my right foot, and says it is a picture. He recognizes it as an instrument of penance that he and the other men used at seminary, to whip themselves on the back with - the blood on my foot looks like a man holding this very instrument.

I ask if I should work today, although I don't know how I can - I can barely stand, and I keep feeling dizzy and the pain is so difficult. He says no, not to work. He tells me to let it go, to not hold onto it, but to transform it, to reflect it back to God. All the while, the whipping occurs, and each time I jump and cry in pain. I try to hold the noise back, but Fr. Francis says it is OK to make sounds. The blood is all poured down between my toes and fingers. The cut on the side makes it difficult because the elastic of my scrubs fits there. I lie down on the couch in my office. What to do with the clients for the day? We give them an option - they can come in and see what is going on, or they can reschedule, or both. Many come, and cry, and feel blessed, and some calls are made to friends and family. All seem moved to faith. I have not much strength, and am glad to lie down.

We find out later that many healings occur at this time, without my even putting my hands on people; that just witnessing the stigmata is a blessing for many. How wonderful, it just goes to show who is In Charge of the healings, He literally has placed His mark upon them, again, there is no doubt Who the real Healer is here.

The bleeding abates, but Fr. Francis says not to wash the area until it coagulates, which it doesn't until the afternoon, which is when it has been the slowest usually. Many photos are taken to document it. I receive food, cards, flowers, prayers and songs in Hebrew, and a cold compress on my forehead. I lie "in state" for visitation until 4pm, and fade in and out at times from the pain. Then two companions gently clean the areas around the wounds, and pour the water out on the Angel statue in front of the Institute, and in a few other places outside. I am driven home, since I cannot drive myself. I cannot eat. Also, for the last three days there has been diarrhea and bouts of fever. My two cats wouldn't come near me, this lasted the three days - they stayed about 4-6 feet away. Then tonight, they start to return to me, getting closer. Also, I start to feel different. In the evening it had always been worse before, now there was only a bit of new blood. I know it is ending. This is the evening of the third day. My mind reflects that Jesus was in the grave three days before his resurrection.

Friday July 22nd

I wake up refreshed, relieved and not bleeding, the wounds are already starting to close up and heal. There is a very strong smell of honeysuckle flowers, so strong it makes my stomach feel nauseated, it lasts several hours. There is no new fluid running from the statues. I start to feel very hungry, but there is no food in the house - I find a ripe avocado outside in the grove, under the trees, and I am able to walk short distances. Today is a day of recuperation, no work to do, and I sleep most of the day. Fr. Francis calls, I tell him *"it is finished."* He is happy for me. I had asked him for contact information to anyone he knows that may know about this, or have experienced it, and he says to keep it close right now, and to wait until I am fully recuperated first. I still need to know for later, since this will happen again. I ask why mine didn't go all the way through, and had it always gone through on others? By not doing the healing on the third day did we prevent it from going further, would it have continued? I don't know.

When I was well, I started doing research. Padre Pio, a modern stigmata-bearer, lasted 50 years, non-stop. Others had their stigmata come and go. In the research, there are 321 total cases in history who have had it, 90% of them are women. How many more were not verified by the Catholic Church, who are in other religions, so weren't counted? How many are there living with it now? I wish there was a way to talk to another person who is experiencing it. I pray for this. This is not something we are prepared for in school! I would like to talk to another who has it, I suppose it is similar to having traveled to another country and wanting to share the adventure with someone who has as well, and to me, this was new country. But truly, my Driver knew the route.

Fr .Francis also tells me he noticed that the potted plant that I gave him for his birthday last week directly dried up and died on the day my stigmata started. Also, he said today he noticed all the same leaves came back from dryness to new green, just like death and resurrection, and it occurred the same time as my suffering ended and my recuperation began, like the resurrection. I think this is another verification for him, besides the unusual picture he recognized on my foot. Today I feel wonderful and happy, and peaceful and tranquil, like I just came back from the Olympic games and have won every medal! It is a wonderful day, and my daughter and her friend bring salmon and steamed vegetables, and more flowers, and I am able to eat a little and rest.

Saturday July 23rd
Today I have almost all my strength back, and the wounds on my hands and feet are now white and only a bit of redness of the skin around the holes. I put the oil from the statues on my scabs to keep them soft. I drive myself without any problems, and wear shoes that leave the wound part exposed on top without being rubbed. I go to the pharmacy with a friend and ask for a salve, and Father tells me to show the pharmacist why. He looks at me and backs away! He seems disgusted and answers me begrudgingly. Oh well, we are always given opportunities to expand each other's faith, and I will do as I am asked. People will accept or reject it on their own; it is not my responsibility. My job is only to make the opportunity, and it does not matter if I am accepted or rejected, for I know who I am in the eyes of God. The wound on

83

my side is a bit more difficult, since I am bending and it is being rubbed by clothes. They are all beginning to itch as they heal. They are healing very fast, and filling in with new material and getting smaller by the hour.

My emotions are relieved that it is over, no more pain, and I have mobility again to come and go as I please. But, I also feel a deep sadness, and really don't want the holes to disappear, since all this really seems surreal. I am actually hoping there will be scars, although from what I have been told, some don't leave any marks. I just don't want to ever forget this moment, I want to see the physical evidence everyday of this wonderful adventure! I make the prayerful request to keep the scars, and am told it will be fulfilled. I look at some of the pictures that were taken on Thursday morning, I usually hate pictures of myself. And here I am without makeup of any kind, and hair a mess. etc. And I realize I look better than I have ever looked in my entire life, because my body is representing Love's body and grace. I get to be a sign-post for signs and wonders – and I am thankful.

I can't wait until the next time, each time. Because each time is new information, and with the new cellular brightening it becomes easier for me to understand the deeper things, ask questions, and get clear, immediate answers. In a way, I am learning to be out of body while still in the body; it is a place of connection and Oneness directly aware and interacting with the All. It truly would take another book to share with you all that *has* been learned, and *continues* to be, so this is an ongoing process for me on my journey, and I am very, very thankful. And all will be shared, since this information is not just for me; information given to one person never is just for that one person, but all persons in the Oneness.

Nothing is held back from me, I and the Father are One, as are you too. (Jn. 10:30) We are all in this together. *Nothing good is held back from any of us.* And together, let us continue to share all that we have learned with one another, even if it sounds unrealistic. Let us continue to become re-created and regenerated in all ways, and become fine instruments of Light in the hands of God, so we can interact fully in a Divine state without restraint of any kind, even while in the body. It's all about Love!

CHAPTER 6

Understanding Time in Remote Viewing & Psychometry
Coding Vibrations for Medical Intuition
& Criminal Investigations

There are records of remote viewing (RV) and its neighbor, the out of body experience (OOBE), throughout all cultures and places throughout time. It was always considered a holy supernatural act, and the remote viewer a person worthy of respect. It has become popular again today, as people continue to brighten and remember who they are and what they can do.

Here's one from the Biblical Old Testament: *"Where have you been, Gehazi?" Elisha asked. "Your servant didn't go anywhere," Gehazi answered. But Elisha said to him, "Was not my spirit with you when the man got down from this chariot to meet you?" (2 Kings 5:26)* And this one from Paul in the New Testament: *"I know a man in Christ who fourteen years ago was caught up to the third heaven. Whether it was in the body or out of the body I do not know - God knows. And I know that this man - whether in the body or apart from the body I do not know, but God knows – was caught up to paradise. He heard inexpressible things..." (2 Cor. 12:1-4)*

Records of other Holy men throughout the world have written and drawn pictures of their experiences too. Yogis and the San call it the "large body" experience, where the person travels out of body and sees his earth body, and perceives it as being huge or elongated. OOBEs have really been a common occurrence throughout history and helps us to recognize the continuity and shared experiences of all cultures and peoples. This includes the awakening to numerous and various healing modalities, including the ability to medically intuit a disease or malady. In this chapter, we choose the best of all worlds, and look at medical intuition (MI) and in the distant healing (DH) relationship.

Medical intuition is not a necessary item to have for healing to occur in a client. But, it can be a welcome tool to convince a client of what is occurring is real. Also, progress of previous healing sessions can be easily seen this way.

However, unless you are a medical doctor you cannot legally give a medical diagnosis, and rightly so. Especially since a "catch 22" can occur - as when a healing happens and changes the original malady. Remote viewing for medical intuition is about learning focused intent, and distant mental interaction with specific targeted knowledge.

Legal Ramifications of Medical Intuition and Healing

Every state in the U.S. has different necessary wordage requirements for the disclaimer paperwork that you and/or your client need to have; but there are some basic points most states want you to address. These include: (1). what training the practitioner has completed; (2). what service is being offered; (3).what benefit can be expected.

The following is only *part* of a "disclaimer," just to give you an idea; please do not use it "as is," since it is incomplete and will not fulfill all the legal requirements that you need:

Please note - participation with Tiffany Snow in a Divine Healing session mandates agreement with the following: A Divine Healing session is not a substitute for medical or psychological diagnosis, and/or for treatment. Tiffany Snow does not diagnose conditions, nor does she prescribe, perform medical treatment, nor prescribe substances, nor interfere with the treatment of a licensed medical professional. The client understands that this Divine Healing session is complementary to healing arts services licensed by the state of California, though these services are not directly licensed by the state itself. Tiffany Snow is not licensed by the state as a healing arts practitioner, but has received certificates in several healing modalities and ministries, along with unique empirical experience. It is recommended that the client see a licensed physician, or licensed health care professional for any physical or psychological aliment he may have.

Customizing Your Skills - What You Need to Know About YOU

Before we focus "out" to remote view for MI, it is necessary to spend ample time "in" for understanding how *you interpret answers* to the questions you seek, and which of your senses are the strongest, and which ones should be more strongly developed. Several of these skills may come together to help you remote view more precisely than you ever imagined. Intuitive self-knowledge is intrinsic to a wide variety of higher mental functions. Start with prayer before doing these things, for you are then requesting strength and power beyond your own, in the Oneness of God everything occurs. In this exercise, seeking simple "Yes" or "No" (Y&N) answers can fine-tune your skills very easily.

"My remote viewing information comes in many ways: symbols, sounds, feeling, tastes, fragments, pictures (accurate and inaccurate), and holistic impressions..." - Mind Trek by Joseph McMoneagle

Seeing - All of our five senses have senses "hidden" behind them. For example, we have our physical sense of seeing with our eyes, but there is also the sense of "seeing" with our mind's eye too - visions, moving pictures, photograph snapshots in our head - the sense of *clairvoyance.* This is my strongest sense, and comes naturally to me, so this is the easiest way for me to use MI. A person can ask the quick Y&N questions and "see" a *red light* for *"No,"* and a *green light* for *"Yes"* in their mind's eye. They can then move very quickly to the problem. When you get there, you can give the intention to "zoom in" and have a screen show the full details of the area, in a photographic layout or video presentation that appears in your. With me, this occurs whether my eyes are open or closed.

Hearing - Some people are more proficient in psychic hearing, or *clairaudience.* Gifted evidence-based mediums such as John Edward, James van Praagh and Allison Dubois have excellent "hearing" skills that they can utilize to receive names, locations, and personal details of the deceased people they contact in their work. Whereas with me, I still see those who have transitioned better than I hear them, so I would describe how they physically look and the scenes they psychically show me of places, people and objects of value in their life. I have to work harder to hear than I do to see, unless it is coming direct from Father. In medical intuition, when you use SPI (specific prayerful intent) for details, if you are more gifted in the audio department, you might audibly *hear* the actual words Y&N in your head for the answers you seek. Or, you may *hear* the actual name of the disease, where a tumor is located, or what mix of medications are causing problems so the doctor can be asked to check for contraindications.

Scent - The sense of smell is delivered immediately to the brain and makes more of an impact than we realize in our daily routine. How many times has an aroma connected you with a treasured memory? The smell of sage and juniper on a high desert in the warmth of the setting sun; the salt spray of the ocean; mom's hot apple pie with cinnamon; the perfume or cologne worn on a first date - all are olfactory joys that can transport the consciousness through time. Without our sense of smell, food also becomes unappealing and separated from previous pleasurable memories related to each dish. For those of you who are aware of the sense of smell, you might sense a *putrid odor* for *"No,"* and a *sweet one* for *"Yes."* Experiment!

Taste - Taste is very closely related to scent - and the same psychic sense seems to apply here as for smell: a *sour* or *bitter taste* for *"No,"* and a *pleasant* or *sweet one* for *"Yes."* Some medications you may also taste when you place your hands on someone. A metallic taste, the toxic taste of the body's reaction to marijuana or other street drugs, or even the taste of wine or hard liquor may be on your tongue as you medically intuit someone.

Feel - This is often called a "gut feeling" by the guys and "women's intuition" by the gals. This can be an actual physical sensation of *sickness, nausea* or *anxiety* when utilized as a "No," and a *highly caffeinated* and *confident feeling* when it is a "Yes." Since *feeling* often encompasses the entire bodily system, it is NOT preferable for frequent and immediate answers in MI. However, it can be an excellent "back-up system" to verify some of the subtle answers you receive. Utilizing your whole body for receiving messages in this way can be draining and may eventually result in a subconscious resentment of the work, because of the strain placed upon your physical system. Using these methods is a touch-stone for our humanness, and should be altered to fit your areas of greater sensitivity as you recognize them.

How to Sense and Observe without Controlling the Outcome

I have found a direct correlation between the desire to control and the problems that many healers and intuitives have with their health. The adrenal response and other factors that are triggered by constant subjection of the system can create havoc - but only if the healer feels responsible for some part of the situation. This is the part of the ego needing to "do something" to control the outcome. This needs to be released in trust to God.

Again, I encourage all senses to pass *"through"* you, and not *"end"* in you. One can be fully aware and a channel of positive light without needing all the answers and influencing all the outcomes. Similar to watching fish in an aquarium, we can choose to observe and watch the sensations swim by, without feeling the need to reach out and manually direct each movement. Our job is to allow the fish to swim where they please, and to better their environment the best we can, with food, warmth, adventurous surroundings and fresh water. And it is up to them to interact within their environment as they wish, and this gives us the freedom to observe without controlling.

With further advancement in spiritual awareness, the healer can come to a place of trust, the true meaning of the word "faith," and be content with the ripple effect of simply holding a constant vigil of peace. No matter what terror and darkness falls around us, we continue to hold up the lighted torch. We don't put the torch down to battle the monster, thereby also stumbling in the darkness and being consumed by fear, but we stand our ground and the monster eventually backs off from the light, as do the shadows themselves. In time we learn this, and it gives us full freedom to love without restraint, and to heal without ego attachment.

Now, you *need* to know what your strengths are, and *practice* them! This will give you confidence in your ability to receive accurate messages. It will also let you identify and develop the weaker senses. The more senses and input you can receive about a subject, the better your MI hit rate will be, and the more beneficial the information provided to the client. Many people start with one sense they are aware of, and end up with two or more operating very well. Remote viewing requires super-sensitivity and super-efficiency. Ingo Swann, often called the "father of remote viewing," compares the mind to a "software" program, a "mental information processing grid." He believes remote viewing occurs by simply converting various forms of input energy to another form the sensory system can read, much like a transducer for information. I agree with him.

Observing without Supposing

In remote viewing, as well as distant healing, we learn to strike a balance between observing, without being emotionally overwrought about the end result. Absolutely knowing in your core that what is received is exactly what is *supposed* to be received, and that it will happen at exactly the *right time* for it, is crucial to letting go of "performance" anxiety. It is this ability to be nonjudgmental that allows the state of full awareness and accuracy in relating events, illnesses and information. This allows the free intention of asking all questions and receiving all information without clogging ourselves up to the answers we may not want to perceive. With practice and experience an advanced intuitive can "tune in" quickly and without much preparation, and expect to produce much better results than the average MI person. Thus, we have learned to tweak our radio channel until we get music for our ears, and how to *ignore most of the static.*

This neutrality to outcome, while still keeping oneself in full balance and complete love for the task at hand can make it difficult to work on friends and family members. When our own emotions are running high, it is hard to "get yourself out of the way," and the results often reflect this. Sometimes we find ourselves pushing in our own energy, and we will feel the consequences in our minds and bodies. In these cases, asking another healer to assist can help us keep our balance.

Especially while participating in research studies, self-implied pressure may create clogging because of fear of failure. This can produce poor results for truly gifted intuitives and healers. Other people's expectations and feedback (for good or bad) should not be allowed to affect your results. Please keep in mind that you are not trying to please anyone, but doing what you must do, the passion of your soul. As you practice and push the boundaries of only your own expectations, keep in mind that none of us are perfect in any of this, and whatever you can do is fine and has benefits. If you desire to go further, then relax and just do it, and it will happen.

"The success of love is in the loving - it is not in the result of loving. Of course it is natural in love to want the best for the other person, but whether it turns out that way or not does not determine the value of what we have done." - Mother Teresa

"Ask and You Shall Receive" with Remote Viewing

As you learn to go into specific prayerful intention (SPI) and center your attention for more prolonged periods, you will have greater clarity and better detail with your remote viewing. If you are setting your SPI and have yet to get an answer, then repeat it again and again until you have better insight. If you have an assistant or proctor available, this is when his suggestions to focus and go deeper, or his repeating the question over again, can help.

In reviewing some remote viewing techniques, please remember these basics:

(1). Formulate the question you want to know
(2). Make sure you have enough interest or motivation in getting the answer.
(3). Concentrate on that question for as long as needed.
(4). Assume you will naturally get the answer.
(5). Drop into a "blank mind" state of expectancy and wait for the
    impressions to come.

Allow your internal consciousness to communicate these "chalk board" impressions through voice or tactile expressions. Passion creates the interest and intensity for all this to happen. If you are not interested in the outcome, the signal path will not be powerful enough to perceive clearly. This is where love of mankind and the gift of helping one another come truly comes to the forefront. Prayer strengthens the signal line. The true desire to help and make a difference will give you motivation enough even when you do not know the persons as individuals.

91

If you are not seeing reasonably sharp and clear pictures, there is not enough in your memory for the signal to access and to give definition. In other words, you can develop greater accuracy through the repeated practice of your ability and feedback of the outcome, and this will hone your skills. But, you have to have something "in there" for the bits of information floating through to stick on and your brain to interpret it to make sense. There needs to be a recognition of sorts, a relationship to memories or personal knowledge, and often these come as subtle cues.

It is similar to the person born blind who can't imagine colors. In the same way, information doesn't make sense if you can't relate it to anything you know. Study your craft so your mind can access the information it needs to give the answers to the questions you want. With MI, you would want to study anatomy. If you want to utilize RV for archeology, you would want to include cartography and ancient civilizations. Become specific in what you have interest in, and your subconscious will be an ample treasure trove for the information it writes on your internal chalk board. This emphasizes why some people are better in their fields of interest than in others, such as sensitives who help with criminal investigations, or those who help the government with intelligence or invisible espionage.

Color-Coding Vibrations for Medical Diagnosis

There are many different methods that work for medical intuition, especially when you're in a hands-on situation with a client in the room with you. In this case, you might *see* clairvoyantly in your mind's eye a mental picture of what is going on or notice different colors appear over different areas of the body. Often, different things will *feel* different under a sensitive hand. There are different vibrational qualities attached to different problems. Remember that Einstein said all matter is "slowed down energy," and the new physics have indeed shown that there really is no "matter" at all, but only energy simply vibrating at different rates. Through time, I have been able to assign colors to different oscillations, in this way making the diseases and ailments much easier to remember. Even with my background of years of composing and playing music, memorizing such a variety of vibrational patterns proved   most difficult; whereas organizing color combinations do not.

At first I didn't know anything at all - I would sense a certain vibration, and find out afterward what it was when the person would say *"I have diabetes,"* or *"I have heart* disease." Then I would keep that vibration in memory and assign it an easy color pattern of up to five colors (i.e. cancer is "orange," AIDS "orange-brown," diabetes "blue-white" etc.) When I felt that same vibration again in someone else, I would softly venture the question, and in this way I learned the accuracy of it and developed an entire color system. Don't be surprised if this assigning a color to a malady facilitates your having immediate diagnosis of an ailment. Even by just shaking a hand, the trained subconscious will then take the vibrations and form the color patterns in your mind, giving you a diagnostic impression.

A Word about Colors - This is Not about Reading Auras

Except for perhaps the *"red light/green light"* that most of us are familiar with because of traffic signals, all colors should be *uniquely* expressed and meaningful to you. In other words, you wouldn't want to use someone else's ideas for what colors mean - you would want to choose to experience that for yourself. Developing sensitivity to color is not difficult, but it does take time to know what that color specifically means to *you*.

It is important to know I'm not talking about the colors of auras here. I have seen that auras change with moods, and that makes them not accurate enough for MI. Even though sometimes dark colors or shadows may seem consistent over a problem area, I suggest that if you see auras that you only use them as a cue to help you focus awareness to that part of the body, and then use your other senses to look deeper.

There are many games that you can play to increase *all* your senses, which I go over in detail in several chapters of my previous book *"Psychic Gifts in the Christian Life - Tools to Connect,"* so I won't go over any of them here. But knowing what colors mean to *you* and games to sharpen sensitivities can trigger an excellent response in the hidden senses when you SPI your questions. By assigning every color with one of the five senses, you will be

93

given that color answer through the sense that is stronger for you, or even through several senses at once! For example: perhaps you have worked with the color *yellow,* and have assigned it to the various senses, finding yellow "tastes" like banana, "smells" lemony, "feels" rubbery, and "sounds" like the song "Yellow Submarine." Now, when your SPI stimulates your stronger senses and wants to give you *yellow* for your answer, you may *taste* banana, *hear* "Yellow Submarine," and so forth, depending on your natural and practiced gifts of discernment.

Why learn colors? Because they go hand-in-hand with vibrations and oscillations. Let's say you have assigned "epilepsy" as yellow. You touch someone, and since you have discovered that you are an *audible* gifted person, you hear your corresponding *yellow* song in your head, perhaps "Good-bye Yellow Brick Road." Now you get the hint, and realize the person you just touched has epilepsy. God has each of us "hard-wired" to receive His impressions through our senses. Life is a color kaleidoscope!

Color Applications for Crime Scene Investigation

Besides the usefulness in a "hands-on" diagnosis, there is also application in utilizing this tool in crime scene and missing person investigations. For example, during SPI you might ask for the color of shirt the perpetrator was wearing or his skin color, if the missing child is dead or alive, etc. All this can be seen by customizing your ability to receive this specialized information.

As we have seen through our foray in the quantum world, once one thing has been in contact with another, there is a connection that affects both, no matter how far apart they are from each other. This is a clue to why holding an object from the scene of a crime, or even a photograph of the victim is most helpful, and also why I ask for a photo or personal information for distant healing. There is an "energy dusting" that allows a target to be related and specifically identified for information to be brought out of the "static" of all other information. This is why it is difficult to target the future, since we don't usually have an indent or location for it, to draw the information out.

Psychometry for Gaining Additional Intuitive Information

Psychometry is reading objects by touch, and generally refers to the ability to gain impressions and information about an object or anything connected to it by holding it in your hand. In 1842 Joseph Buchanan, an American physiologist, coined the term and claimed it could be used to measure the "soul" of all things, and that "the past is entombed in the present."

He theorized that everything gave off an energy emanation that recorded the emotional history of the object, which then played back in the mind of the person holding the object. Impressions from the object will always come in the form recognized by our five senses - which happen to be the same ones we have already indicated - sounds, scents, tastes, pictures or feelings.

With psychometry, we are using the tangible object as a touch-stone for accessing intangible information, and then bringing it into our energetic field to manifest as a message we can understand. This is another method of contact to the "Ultimate Observer," the scientific term and description often recognizable by many as the source of all knowledge and wisdom, the place-holder of the unified consciousness of the mind of God. Wisdom can be thought of as the mind of God revealed. *"If any of you lacks wisdom, he should ask God, who gives generously to all without finding fault, and it will be given to him."* (James 1:5)

Understanding Time and Specifying a Date

Being specific about *time* is important. When the mind accesses information, it accesses not just the present, but future and past. In your SPI, you must remember to specify what *time period* you wish information for. This helps focus and narrow the intent to a narrow time frame. And this is why I ask for a *date of birth* for which I am seeking healing and medical intuition, or the *date of the crime* from investigators and detectives.

In my out of body travels, I have seen time flow like water in a stream, whose rivulets lead to larger rivers, which then moves into deeper ocean pockets. I have seen time speed up and slow down, and even puddle in places. Perhaps this can be likened to what some physicists have implied by M-theory, which involves eleven spacetime dimensions. In my experience, there are more than eleven - and time has the ability to interconnect, bend and circle to wherever it wishes, and definitely does not move along in straight linear path. The extra spatial dimensions of string theory allow for time to curl up, and they exist everywhere.

I have seen *time* to be an inaccurate measurement and weak invention of mankind. Time did not exist before man's creation on this planet, it is only a frail concept for the mind of man to identify a beginning and end according to his own reference of reality. In the bigger sense of things, there is no time, or rather, there is timelessness, or time indefinite. And each of us has that "knowing" and wonderment of eternity in our very spirit. Everything we see around us has a beginning and an end. Even the tallest redwood trees, which live to be hundreds of years old, still live and die. The rocks even had a beginning. Everything around us is in a form of transition, which makes sense, since even matter at its core is only moving energy and not stagnate or "dense" at all. And as I had mentioned earlier, since mankind can only identify that which he can make reference to in his brain, he can only respond to those memories and stimuli in an incomplete way. Such it is for referencing time.

The awakening of healing, and intuitive abilities that many have is because *we now have an information signal for the memory to access and define* beyond the color-blindness we were born into. The veil has been lifted, if even for a moment, and a paradigm of new possibilities can be intentionally manifested as new realities, beyond any restriction of time and space. We have those empirical bits of information sticking to our brain - aiding, sorting and interpreting our experiences in a brand new way. Our brains are "rewiring" new relationships to how we sense and perceive all things, including our knowledge of our relationship to the Oneness. Thus, we awaken to abilities and awareness we never thought possible before.

CHAPTER 7

Advanced Sensory Remote Viewing
for Medical Intuition
How to Do It - Original Methods You Can Chart & Customize

Since we are spiritual beings living in physical bodies, a physical connection aids us in balancing ourselves between both worlds. This is the same sacred place that ritual has occupied for thousands of years in all corners of the earth. It also continues to today in various forms, including those in many religious traditions. We give a wedding ring to symbolize our never-ending love. We wear a cross to feel connected to values and ideals we hold dear. We carry a photo of our departed friend to remember and feel him close.

To gather tangible information from an invisible realm, you can add a tangible item as an aid to keeping this balance. Purchase a medium size teddy bear. Besides grounding you, this will help your medical intuitive ability to seamlessly move intention from one part of the body to another, without having to interrupt the flow with wondering what to look at next. It should have a large enough body to place your hands easily under its neck, to differentiate solar plexus from thoracic cavity, and also have relaxed arms and legs. Sewn eyes are preferable to plastic ones, which can distract because of the coldness felt when working over the eyes. Short snouts are preferable to long ones, with sewn noses for the same reason.

It is not recommended to use a doll since it colors the perception of the sex of the distant healing client, since we have already perceived in our mind the doll as female. The teddy bear should be a new item, and not have any emotional attachments from your childhood, etc, that could influence your RV. It should only be used in MI and DH sessions, and put away afterward, out of sight. This is a sacred tool unlike any other, and should be treated as such, and not get any other "vibes" on it from unwanted comments or people touching it, since you are in a heightened place of awareness when you are using this tool.

It is also not recommended to use your own personal body as a stand-in for the person you are healing. This can be dangerous. Often it is hard to separate what *we* are feeling from what the *client* is feeling, especially if it is for a sustained period of time, such as in a healing session. It is not recommended.

What *is* recommended, is purchasing an anatomical chart, which lets you know without a doubt what you are looking at, or taking classes in anatomy, or viewing any learning course DVDs about the human body. All these things can then be brought back to your mind during the medical intuition process. Using the chart along with the bear is a good idea.

Before you start, there are a few things that you should have already received. The target information of first and last name, age and birth date, town, and country; and perhaps even a photograph. Have this information ready to review, and prime it into your tape recorder if you are using one. Turn off your phone and remove any possible distractions, including Junior and Fluffy (children and pets).

First the Remote Viewing Medical Intuition, *then* the Distant Healing

I am supposing that you will be doing the healing right after the remote viewing, so preparation for an out of body experience (OOBE) is necessary at this first step to have everything prepared for the second. Empty your bladder, have pillows propped and enough clothes or a blanket to keep you warm but not overly so. Being too warm will put you to sleep! Put a new tape in the recorder, or make sure your secretary or assistant is also comfortable if you are using one. This includes him having what tools are needed for note taking, and knowing where to put the disk or paper when he is done. After you finish the remote viewing part of the healing and move into the distant healing phase, you won't be talking anymore, so unless you want to add additional information after you return from DH, they can excuse themselves quietly and leave.

Remember that the *remote viewing intuitive* work needs you to have conscious use of your body to talk, draw, etc. This is the terrestrial, "in" the body work. But for the advanced *out of body distant healing* technique, it is celestial work, fully "out" of the body.

98

Easy Medical Intuition Step by Step

(1). Coordinate the intuitive and healing time to occur while the client is *asleep*. The 10% of our brain acts as a bridge or barrier to the possibilities of healing, so having the client asleep puts to rest any thought of *"I wonder if this is working?"* or *"am I feeling anything happening?"* This opens many unnecessary barriers and clogging, as long as the Free Will of the client has decided to participate in the first place.

Keeping a world time zone chart available will help you know the hours of difference between the both of you. Look at the United States or World map and see where your client is located, so you can "see" approximately where they are. Have your specific intention set for "real-time," to know what is happening now with the client, not the future or past, while you ask for the medical intuition or other questions for which you are looking.

I always try to SPI for future and past information also, but it is a good idea to make a *separate* intention of it, and work on one level of your job at a time. For example, you may want to look at the physical body first, then the emotional overlay and any spiritual things that come up after that. Many times in these levels you will be given past knowledge on how the injuries occurred, or see a number or date related to it, or an internal video of the information. This often happens for the personal validation of the client, for them to remember and understand the relationship between an experience (cause) and outcome (effect). You are there to help them remember who they are, and to receive and identify information that has remained hidden or been buried over time, and to bring them an opportunity to own it, or release it. You are there to be a place of access to the new physics of possibilities in the holographic mind of God.

(2). Create a sacred space for your own quiet and calmness, and pray for no less than 20 minutes before the healing time. This opens one ear to heaven and one to earth. There is a melding inside, and outside, into One, which includes you and the person to be healed. This is similar to quantum superposition, which is being in one or more places at once, by experiencing many

99

possibilities at one time, and then collapsing onto one, which would be your specific intention - either with DH or MI.

Make sure you haven't had over-stimulating sensory awareness beforehand such as arguments or excitement, road-rage traffic, TV or movie, or caffeine. Unless you are very able to "turn off the volume," many of these things will create noise in the mind, asking for resolving, decision making, or replay. These things can too easily creep into the blank state and "muddy the waters" of remote viewing. In this state, you might think something of your own making is theirs, when it definitely is not. Stimulants can make it difficult to calm and focus; and heavy eating can make you fall asleep.

(3). Now, read over the target information, or have your secretary read it out loud. It is your choice to be where you are comfortable and able to focus without distraction. At the institute, I have a red velvet antique "fainting couch" (now re-christianed "prayer couch") where I have a variety of pillows to prop me at a comfortable angle. Across from me is a small marble writing table and stained-glass Tiffany lamp with a soft low-light bulb, just enough illumination to reduce eyestrain for the secretary using the laptop. The dimmer control for the ceiling fan I keep close at hand, to adjust the breeze if I get too hot, which often happens during sessions. I also have a sacred space, a small covered altar in the corner of the room, since I personally choose to offer communion before I work. There is always a glass of water waiting for me after the session. Most of the time I have chosen to do all my work at the Institute, and my fun OOBEs at home.

(4). Recline or lie down, and take the photo and target information and hold it briefly between your hands, and as you quiet your mind start your specific prayerful intent. Now place the target information on your chest or belly. Then hold the teddy bear laying face-up on your solar plexus, with your hands on its head. Since this is an advanced book, I am assuming you have read about or have utilized remote viewing before, and have built the confidence that it works. Now from this place of information and mental clarity, you can customize your RV by sensing all the abilities that work for you.

Perhaps you utilize a blank white screen in your mind's eye, and you look for

100

it to fill it with information. In that same mind's eye, you can see your hands on the person's head. And in your real physical life, your hands are already upon the bear's head. Start asking the questions you need to know, and check all your senses for feedback. Here is where you will see red light / green light for *"yes"* and *"no,"* or any of the other senses you have trained will now kick in. Your hands may get warm, hot or vibrate on the bear, as additional validation indicating where there is a problem. The teddy bear is a simple way to flow a very accurate RV session for medical intuition.

(5). Now, move your hands over the eyes, then nose, mouth of the bear - always asking yourself the simple Y&N questions. Move down the shoulders to the elbows, wrists, and down the hands, being sure to check all the structural joints. Move from the neck down to the heart and out to the lungs, to the stomach, then over to the liver, looking at the different systems and soft organs as you move down the intestines, reproductive organs, hips, knees, ankles and feet.

When you are done with the front part of the body, turn the bear over, and start at the head and again move down the arms, spine, etc. Keep mindful of where your hands are getting hot, and focus your intention over those areas. As you learn to receive better, you will usually find that you will have a "heads-up" even when you first place your hands on the forehead of the bear, because your mind can already see how Spirit is flowing through the body and flooding the areas where it needs to work, before you even get there.

If you have trained yourself with colors, you might see in your mind's eye various diseases or maladies that are presenting. All the while, you are able to talk out loud, since you have control of your body in your terrestrial state. You will be stating whatever you see, including any symbols and thoughts that pass through your mind. If you are able to sketch, you can do this also. It is important to not "figure it out" or to make sense of the things or fit them together somehow. Just state everything as you are presented it, and vocalize it slowly and clearly. First impressions are usually the most accurate, and help keep the analytical mind out of it. Generally, this form of MI RV only lasts 30 - 45 minutes, it is important not to get "hung up" on things, as there are two parts to this process, and you need time for the distant healing too.

Be totally "neutral" in what you get - you are looking for truth, and any thought of "what should be" will color the information. With remote viewing, you are basically 50/50 with still being "in" your body, yet focusing outside of it. This ability to focus and use your brain can easily lend itself to describing the room, the house, many other life-forces living there, etc. You can throw in a few other things as well, which will verify "You were there" to the client - like the layout of the furniture, where the windows are placed, sometimes the color of the curtains or wallpaper.

If you are fairly new to remote viewing, you might find that older furniture is easier to notice than new stuff - I think it is because it has more energy dusting attracted to it; so many emotions spilling out over it through time. So, you might note grandma's antique dresser, yet not the new recliner in the corner. It is "onion layers" of perception that may become clearer in time and usage.

Since my last near-death experience, during the out of body phase I have been able to physically move light-weight objects as well, such as turning spice containers upside down, or folding clothes, etc., which is fun for me, and verifies my presence and helps to expand the client's mind of us being more than a physical body. I often do healings on the animals too, which can always see me, and some of them wake their masters up to tell them so! When you have completed the remote viewing, you can choose to come more fully back into control of your senses and close, and to take a bit of a break between gathering information and "clicking out" for distant healing. Get a glass of water, use the facilities, say good-night to your secretary; you have completed phase one, the medical intuition, and can email the notes the next day to your client.

Setting up Identifiers for *Advanced* Medical Intuition

As we have seen and experienced, remote viewing is the practice of extending our consciousness beyond our body, to observe an event or target somewhere else. Since we are dealing with a client who has requested a viewing and/or a healing, there is a certain amount of "front-loading" that occurs. We are usually given information about a need beforehand. I do not see this as being a negative methodology, although it goes against the strict protocol of RV, since there is no one blind to the target, which is the number one dictate for remote viewing. With medical intuition, I also suggest to the client that he share with me whatever his concerns are, so I am certain to look more closely at that area and spend more time there, for a focused heightened awareness of receiving information. I have discovered that *the ability to correctly assess a problem is not related to the ability to heal it.* It is good to keep in mind these are two different things.

For advanced MI, you first need to set up a consistent identifier, sometimes called a *task number* or *task cue* for the coordinates of the target or objective, which in this case is a human being. Now you are going to take the date of the viewing and the client's birth date as his unique target number. For example, my birthday is January 11th 1962, or 01111962. If I were being remote viewed on Dec. 18th 2006, or 12182006, the combined number of the date of the viewing and my birth date would indent this target as: 1218200601111962, or 12182006-01111962. Or, as I like to do, by using only the last two digits of the birth year, you will still be specific but the number not as long: 121806-011162. For archive purposes, putting the client's birth date first aids in finding the file again, and I use the last name as well (ex. "SNOW 011162-121806"). This is a simple way to make a unique number for each client. In this advanced stage, you will need a drawing pad, pencils, and a copy of the chart I will give you or a chart you have made on your own.

I suggest you set up an identifier even if you feel you know the target well and have worked it before. This aids in archival filing, and works even if it's the same person or place viewed at another time, since the second viewing date would mark a different number. Please keep in mind the following is *not protocol,* but *varied methodologies* for remote viewing.

If you strictly wish to use RV protocol, you can simply set up the identifier the same way as you would any other target - by making sure nobody in the room with or in contact with the viewer (you) at the time of the session knows anything about the target. If the person sitting across the table from you knows the target, it isn't RV. Either way, when you suggest after a RV that the client then goes and gets medical diagnosis, this will be feedback for you - though often you will find they already knew about their problem, or had a "hunch" about it. But one of the nice things about what we are doing is that we don't stop with just looking at the problem, but combine it with distant healing, which allows The Big Guy to do something about it!

Not There Yet – But Deeper Still

(1). As previously stated, I suggest that the medical intuition and distant healing occur while the person is asleep, you know his time zone and location, and have set your intention for "real-time," to know what is happening now with the client. If the future or past is important to the outcome of the healing, then take the time to specifically intention that further along in your session. It really is good to separate it out when you are dealing with aspects of time.

(2). Create a sacred space for quiet and calmness. Use this as an additional time for cool down before you work. This is a time to physically relax, and emotionally to become centered, emptying the mind of any preconceptions. If you wish to further create a ritual that aids in your relaxation, such as lighting a candle, or listening to your favorite song, then go ahead. Any preparation is to help suspend your disbelief, to open to supernatural awareness, to be confident in the new adventure on which you are about to embark. It is about being God-aware and realizing how powerful a person and well-connected you are to all things. In the beginning, some might want to start their remote viewing or distant healing by reading stories ahead of time that help facilitate the attitude of full acceptance of this experience. The more advanced you become and the more results you see, the less time you will need to tell your analytic brain that all this is OK to do and very real, because you will be living beyond the common reality and *absolutely know it as an undeniable fact.*

(3). Write the target number (birth and healing date) at the top of your page. It is still your choice to either read over the full target material given by the client, or not. This can include specific concerns they may have about physical health, future events, releasing past traumas, contacting dead loved ones, or requesting words of knowledge from God. I personally believe and trust in being fully open to whatever information I am presented, and going into the situation entirely open. I also think reviewing the material helps center me on the actual target. My job is not to judge or interpret, but to simply present what I see to the best of my ability. Any and all interpretation is up to the client. And if there is something specific I can address for him, all the better incentive to look for the answer.

(4). Become comfortable in a place where you can draw easily in your terrestrial state, and place beside your drawing pad an anatomical chart for clearer focus. Perhaps you like using clay for three-dimensional work, such as showing a tumor on a kidney. Clay utilizes both hands, keeping the RVing brain balanced, and often gives additional depth and dimension that a sketch pad cannot, although it takes a higher awareness to utilize in the altered state.

Start your SPI, and further cool your mind to a place of clarity and calm. Have your assistant write the identifier at the top of his page too. It is a good idea to have a monitor, or a liaison person to guide your intentions and refocus your direction if you go too deep. If you start to lose the terrestrial connection, they can bring you back from the edge of consciousness by tasking the questions.

In my case, an assistant can also keep me from getting lost in the person's dreams, or their recurring thoughts, which I see and feel while I am with them, and can distract me and lead me into many tangents which may not be necessary or beneficial. Sometimes these dreams and thoughts aid me in knowing what the emotional aspect is to the presenting malady, and I will state it in my notes to them. As a successful remote viewer, you want to continue fully in a self-trance state, the place between awake and asleep, called the hypnagogic state. At least until you are ready to go to the next step, which is the OOB distant healing.

For me, the most difficult part of viewing is consciously moving body parts other than my mouth. Moving my hands to sketch is energetically stressful for me, yet I understand the valuable information only gathered here. It is a place of continual practice for me, since especially in criminal investigations and missing person cases drawing a location map, etc., is important.

105

Also, in the beginning a student may be responding to the assistant's questions, yet answering him only in his head, while thinking he is moving his lips and being audibly heard! More experience insures a greater ability to get to the edge of consciousness, without falling over. Also in time, if you use a consistent monitor, they too will know and sense when to pull you back in and re-direct you.

Note Taking and Sketching

Once you have relaxed into the receptive state, you can "prime the pump" by looking at the things you were already told, to simply verify that they exist. After you can describe the basic elements, the monitor can then pose further questions about the target, and write down what you say. Leave all the writing up to him - you are using your paper only for sketching. After the session, you can review the notes and write in anything to help clarify what was perceived.

Especially in criminal cases, I have *already written out* the questions that the detectives have asked. I give these to the monitor to task me, after he recognizes (or I tell him) that I am in a highly receptive state and ready to get the information.

So after I arrange myself comfortably, I bring myself up to the level of peace, and clarity of mind. After 8-10 minutes, my assistant will start speaking, if I have not, and he will ask the first question. I always want the first question to be one asking if I have acquired the target. It might go like this: "We are looking for the body of Matthew M., do you see him?" If I respond in the affirmative, we can go on. If it's, "no, I don't see him," then my assistant knows to wait another 4 or 5 minutes and ask the question again. Most of the time I get a hit right off, but rarely it can take me up to three times. I have yet to fail to acquire a target, though accuracy can fluctuate for a variety of reasons.

I wait for any casual information to come, and make notation of it - symbols, thoughts, any impressions from my senses, etc. I speak any words out loud, and often incoherently explain what I am drawing, without implying or supposing (this is why it is chaotic, but it helps me to ramble with the drawing

106

- it may or may not help for you). I try to keep all my senses awake and available for impressions. You might want to experiment with breathing to get you further into "the zone," faster, deeper, shallower or slower - have fun with it. Like a scuba diver adjusting the air in his BC jacket for optimum buoyancy, this will adjust your attention and relaxation levels and give you more control of the experience. Remember to always start with prayer.

Good-bye Teddy Bear! Customizing and Charting Your Senses

Remember how we used the bear and anatomical chart together previously? Now, you are *not* going to use them, but only a customized chart that you make yourself. This will accord the senses that you have trained the most highly to make themselves known. We are now going to look at several aspects in one chart, which can aid us to individually perceive our answers. Also remember to periodically upgrade and further customize your chart as your other senses come into further development. These charts are only a guideline, an incentive for your own ingenuity and receive-ability.

If you have more than one strong sense, it will help you further organize your experience. Let's say you are strong with Visual and Audio. You could then assign physical problems with colors, and emotional with sounds. Or, sorting it out as you wish, structural problems (bones, etc.) with tones, and soft tissue with color. The variety of your chart can be as varied as you. I do suggest when you first start, to have patience with yourself until you have trained the subconscious response to trigger the color, sound, smell, feeling, or taste for which you are looking. You can do the same thing with crime scenes. For example, I instantly feel physically nauseated when there has been a murder, and by paying attention to that, I can allow my focus to adjust to that area and not waste valuable time in another one.

We are "hard-wired" to receive messages and information from beyond our natural state. Here are some trigger parameters to use for manifesting the hidden senses behind the senses for your own maximum conscious and unconscious responses: *remember to use them simply and consistently without changing their meanings.* For example, if you are EYES/VISUAL, do not color-code every organ, but to choose a color that represents health for all the organs, and to use combinations only for representations of an illness.

Eyes: Seeing/Visual - COLORS. PICTURES. Is a healthy organ *red* to you? Or are you going to assign *red* as a danger color warranting further focus? Does *white* mean free of toxins, or no circulation to that part of the body? Be consistent in your color choices, and soon the entire human body will become beautiful artwork painted before your very (mind's) eyes. Or, you could see an entire photo display or video play inside your head. Visual is one of the best methods for medical intuition.

Ears: Hearing - MUSIC GENRE, TONES/NOTES OR WORDS. You can choose to hear classical music in your mind when a body is orderly and healthy. Or hard rock music when there are drugs in the system Or, maybe you know a bit about the composition of music itself, and choose to set "middle C" as a tone for perfect health, and the corresponding notes that fall above or below show the measure of how out-of-balance that area is. Perhaps intuitively hearing a bird sing means one thing, while a blaring car horn means another - you can use different sounds for different maladies. Or, perhaps you simply hear a voice in your head that tells you exactly what is going on, or gives you Y&N answers to your questions.

Mouth: Taste - SWEET, SOUR, BITTER OR PUNGENT. OR SPECIFIC INDIVDUAL TASTES. You could be given Y&N by two *contrasting tastes* of your choosing. Or, you could choose to not taste anything at all until you come across a problem area. You could also choose individual tastes for specific illnesses, similar to how COLOR is used. Perhaps you taste metallic when the person has cancer, perhaps cinnamon if he is diabetic. You are the one setting the parameters for this, use your imagination.

Nose: Smell - GOOD, BAD, SPECIFIC SMELLS. You could be given Y&N by two *contrasting odors* of your choosing. Or, you could choose to not smell anything at all until you come across a problem area. If you are really up on your olfactory joys, you could even differentiate odors like suggested for Mouth/Taste. The multi-million dollar perfume industry knows the importance of smell to influence moods and thoughts. Find out what various scents mean to you.

Skin: Feel - NAUSEATED, DIZZY, EXCITED, CALM. This is the sense that most people feel they have, but also where you can get out of balance the fastest. By constantly absorbing the energy around you, your own mind and body takes a beating 24/7, and you can end up not knowing what is "theirs," and what is "yours." I suggest that the only aspect of the SKIN sensation you use regularly is the GUT FEELING/WOMAN'S INTUITION for simple Y&N answers, and let your body and mind take a rest from everything else. On occasion and for short periods of time I will ask to feel what the person feels like, if I am having a hard time locating a problem, or if I need further clarification between physical and emotional overlays. But, I don't allow it for long, and neither should you. We are there to help the situation, not to take the problems upon ourselves. We are there to set the pace, not to get run down and run over.

Here are some suggestions for what your chart might look like. I have placed only two sensory aspects in (SEE and HEAR), but you will want to replace these modalities with the ones that are the strongest for you:

SAMPLE CHART

(write your identifier number here – ex. "SNOW 011162-121806")

See WHITE, healthy - Tone Low and relaxed - Smell roses - Taste sweet lemonade
See BLACK , unhealthy - Tone high shrill - Smell moth balls - Taste licorice

Look at the 7 Major Systems:

010 * Brain (cerebellum, cerebral hemispheres) PURPLE=Tone Low DO

020 * Head (head including neck, thyroid,
eyes, ears, pituitary, sinuses, teeth)   BLUE = Tone RE

030 * Chest (lungs, diaphragm,
heart including cardiovascular system)   GREEN=Tone ME

040 * Endocrine (chemical/hormone - pituitary,
hypothalamus, thyroid, adrenals, kidneys, pancreas.
Testes and ovaries from a hormonal aspect)   YELLOW=Tone FA

050 * Digestive (liver, spleen, stomach, gall bladder,
all organs including small and descending intestines) ORANGE=Tone SO

060 * Reproductive (bladder, kidneys, prostate, uterus, urethra,
rectum. Testes and ovaries from a structural aspect)   RED=Tone LA

070 * Lymph (the entire lymphatic system)   PINK=Tone TI

*Please note that the respiratory system will not be evaluated separately, but
at its own placement within the 7 major systems.*

Look at the 3 Basic Systems:

0X * Structure   = Tone Bass Drum
Bone - (blood, arthritis, breaks, osteoporosis)
Spine - (cervical, thoracic, lumbar, sacrum)
Legs - (hip, knee, ankle, foot)
Arms - (shoulder, elbow, wrist, hand)
Flesh - (skin, muscles, tendons, breasts, posterior)

0Y * Nervous System (cranial nerves and spinal cord to hands
and feet)   = Tone Violin

0Z * Emotional & Spiritual   = Tone Piano
Mind - (headaches, recurring memories, trauma, anxiety)
Heart - (relationships, doubt, hopes, dreams)
Throat - (victim, not speaking out,)
Hands - (unfulfilled talents, purpose)

Solar Plexus - (unresolved anger, repression, rage, finances)
Sexual - (sense of loss, abuse, anger, victim, guilt, control issues)

Ways to Use the Chart for Full Intuitive Access

You can use this chart in many ways. It is all about developing your sensitivities in the best way you can. What is the easiest way for the Almighty Oneness of the universe to connect with you? Let's say you can perceive colors the easiest. Even with the chart, there are basic simple ways to work, and more detailed ones. You can make copies of your chart and circle the things you are observing, use it to cue yourself questions, etc.

Simple Example of Seeing: After you have the target in mind, you intent that the colors on the chart reflect PHYSICAL healthy colors for that area. If you see WHITE, the answer is *"Yes."* Remember we are still using basic *"Yes"* and *"No"* to get to the answers. This gives an indication that the problem may have to do with *emotional or spiritual* problems, so you can play the Y&N game with black and white.

Variation: Another way of Seeing is to acquire the target, and intent the colors on the chart as a tool to manifest an *unhealthy* physical system in the body. This could appear as a swatch of color in your mind, or the shape of the organ itself. This occurs when you have trained your mind to set *that* color with *that* organ. For example, as I RV the identifier, I see the color purple, and then know the brain has a problem, and can seek more information on this part of the body. The swatch method is not as accurate as seeing a combination of color with the shape of the organ, since illness might be affecting more than one system at a time, and you wouldn't know it. I also like to take every opportunity to make intention and ask for wellness, and then everything will look good except the parts that aren't in good shape. Then I can work on those.

Constantly asking to see the unhealthiness appear in a body seems energetically too draining for me. I feel it is a higher energy to see the body as whole and balanced, until the unhealthiness presents itself differently from that. It might be compared to a mother looking for the child who ate the family dessert before dinner - mom could line up all the children, tell them they are all bad and will face punishment unless they tell on the one who did it, and thereby instill low vibration and fear into the entire situation. Or, the mother could casually invite everyone to sit down at dinner as usual, and then observe who is too full to eat, and take that one aside for private discussion.

Depending on what sensitivities are your strongest, you can customize your chart as you progress. If you know the shape and location of organs in the body, so much the better. Remember we have to *put information in the brain* before it can be found and *pulled back out again.* I can't emphasize enough about getting a large anatomy chart and becoming very familiar with the shapes, placement and sizes of the organs. With that information in your head, there's a good chance that the problem area will pop up in your mind's eye. You might find some very good resources that are large and simple through education supply houses. There are even some models of men and women who you can piece together for hands-on experience. There are college textbooks with good overlays and drawings. I have greatly benefited from the Teaching Company DVD courses on "Understanding the Human Body: An Introduction to Anatomy and Physiology," presented by Professor Anthony Goodman, M.D. at the Montana State University. They are expensive but well worth the cost for building your accuracy and information level to be accessed later. You are not only investing in your own future, but changing the future of many that are helped by you.

A Fun Exercise with Strict Protocol

If you want to use strict protocol with your remote viewing, make a target pool of identifiers. You will have to be totally blind to the target, so you will need to go through the necessary steps of having other people help you. A pool can be created from an assistant cutting up an old medical textbook, one with pictures of diseases and maladies. These are then sealed in separate envelopes, with a random number generated and applied to the outside of each one. These are then placed into a large manila envelope or box. In a formal exercise, the person who creates the target pool does not participate beyond that. I suggest a minimum of 30 different envelopes. They can be entered back

112

into the pool and used again, but the larger the pool the better, to prevent overlays with the viewer.

When you go about your session, have your secretary reach in and get an envelope. He will then write the identifier number down, and so should you. Allow yourself to experiment with holding the envelope versus having it placed on the table beside you, so you can fine-tune what works best for you without compromising the situation. Your secretary can ask you: "tell me what disease needs to be healed and where it is found on the body," so you can get the disease and the organ, which will both be on the photo. Continue the session like any other session, including speaking out-loud what you see.

Afterward, give your drawings, chart, clay or whatever you have chosen to utilize for gathering information, to the secretary to review and compare with the notes. Or, to make it even more formal an experiment, bring in another person in, in an analyst capacity to compare your information to several open envelopes (including the right one), and see if your accuracy level is high enough for him to identify the right one from your results. Have fun!

Remote Viewing Emotional States

Often, besides the physical, you will receive information about emotional issues, perhaps even with accompanying pictures of the traumatic scenes unfolding in your mind. Sometimes it's previous childhood issues, or a currently unfolding relationship pain. It can be a varied host of previously buried problems that need surfacing to heal. Often when we bury these traumatic things deep inside they fester - and they can cause physical problems as a by-product (science has proven the link between physical and emotional health). *Your job as the remote viewer* is to acknowledge and relate any information you receive. This gives an opportunity for further awareness on the part of the individual, which is often the first step to changing the situation. But *your job as a distant healer* goes farther than this, and will be addressed in the next chapter.

CHAPTER 8

An Honest Appraisal - Are You a Healer?
Eight Questions to Ask Yourself

"Healing" comes in many terms and with many methods; some are hands-on modalities, while some do not touch the body at all. But all are being studied, and the results are good enough to keep millions of people coming back for more. Yes, some techniques and practitioners work better than others do, and this is the case for distant healing too. Distant healing is also called by different names, such as remote healing, nonlocal healing or distant mental influence. Most researchers agree that the most common trait among distant healers is an *"ability to hold a compassionate intention for another at a distance."*

Once again, the capacity for *love* is the integral part of successful distant healing, and is especially true to activate the compassion needed for a person we've never met or seen. It doesn't matter if the person isn't in the room with us, or even in the same country. In a very real way, no healing is distant healing, because we are not "distant" from anybody or anything in our wonderfully entangled quantum world. When we live in the great mystical realization that we are *already* connected together in this matrix of power and Love, we do what we can; what we were built to do. And what we do becomes the incredible…then the incredible becomes miraculous…the miraculous becomes commonplace…and the commonplace becomes a *daily miraculous realization of new realities.*

"We conclude that an individual is indeed able to directly, remotely, and mentally influence the physiological activity of another person through means other than the usual sensorimotor channels…[the second] explanation of our obtained effects is that mind is nonlocal and that under special conditions its non local nature is manifested. According to this view, energy or information does not "travel" from one place to another or from one mind to another, but is already "everywhere." The influencer's mind and the subject's mind may not really be as distinct, separate, and isolated as they

appear to be but, rather, may be profoundly interconnected, unified, omnipresent, and omniscient. What is available to one mind may be available to all minds and may already be part of all minds in what is analogous to a "holographic" form." – Distant Mental Influence by William Braud, Ph.D.

There are more and more research studies available now - a good search on the internet will bring up quite a few universities, informative books, completed data and projects in process. This book is not going to list here what you could read elsewhere, or have already read. We will be simply focused on one specific modality for distant healing that I have found to be extremely successful - the connection of SPI combined with an out-of-body state for miraculous healings.

A Few Testimonies for Distant Healing

"Thank you Tiffany again and again! I now have freedom of movement in my neck and the bones no longer crack and pop. I can move my head to the left and to the right and there is no noise whatsoever! These problems have been bothering me for about 12 years, since the car accident – now they are gone! The day after you worked on me, when I woke up I felt different. Later that day I was riding along with my husband and son and I discovered that I could move my head and neck back and forth and up and down with no cracking and popping anymore...The heaviness in my head was gone. I started to cry tears of joy and I asked my husband if he knew why I was crying and he started guessing everything else. Then I moved my head to let him see. I told him I had been healed, we are so happy! I am truly thankful to God and to you. Miracles are still happening in 2004. I know because it has happened to me, and at a distance too! - A.B., Ohio"

"Tiffany, just wanted to tell you some news you will like to hear. Today O.B. woke up!"(coma client, less than two days after distant healing).

"Many Thanks, Tiffany! As you know, I had a problem with choking, going all the way back to childhood. I was afraid to eat in public or at restaurants, or sometimes even when I was just at home and anxious. I found it very embarrassing. You did the long-distance healing before I got on the plane to

Buenos Aires, I wanted a good vacation with my husband, and to eat on the plane, and on the trip. I just got back. It was great! Managed to eat, not perfectly, but managed fruit and salads and ice cream. My stomach is much better – I'm glad about that, really glad! Very Warmly, - R. G., England"

"Tiffany, I didn't feel anything different after the healing time. I told you I didn't think anything happened. Well, here I am three weeks later, with egg on my face! You won't believe it – well, I know YOU will. The tests came back. You are the only new thing I did. MY RECTAL CANCER IS GONE!!! I will never doubt God again, or you! Forgive me! I'm going to LIVE!!! C.O., Florida"

"You are exactly correct...the medical information is everything that the doctors said, you confirmed it...The emotion/mental notes were too much for me, and it took all day to read, because I kept stopping to cry. I CRIED! I never cry. There was no way you could have known about me from anyone. It made me realize someone (The BIG GUY as you say) was helping you to reach my heart and to get past those things I still had in there, the things that hurt...I feel better today. God bless you and keep you. - D.L., Canada"

"I am sorry for contacting you again, but I wanted to thank you and Jesus for helping with my wife's case. As you know, she could not tell us what was hurting because of all the tubes in her mouth and the damage to her throat. Her temperature was so high, we knew she was still fighting infection, but the doctors couldn't find anything else and didn't want to go back in for more surgery because of her weakness. When you told me what you saw, when you came in and floated on the ceiling and looked, I knew you really did see everything, because you described the nurses so well. Especially the short one with short brown hair whose name began with "T," you were right, she did tell the other nurses my wife was going to die! I really got mad at that, I could sue the hospital, but I won't. I can't have that around my wife. Thank you for letting me know. Also, we are testing where you said to look - she is feeling better today, but for two days after you were here, it was bad, like you said it would be, and now things are getting better, like you said it would be...thanx again. - E.N., California"

"I have never had such a quick diagnosis for a condition...you are exactly right, the tests just came back this morning about dad's heart. It was the same thing you said and you were only a little off on the blood pressure and right on with the cholesterol. Thought I would tell you...they are scheduling the surgery in two weeks..." (one week later) *"...Tiffany, I had a really hard time getting them to do the tests again, but you would never guess! The doctors are saying they want to wait and do more tests, because they can't figure it out, everything has changed. I will tell dad about the distant healing you gave him, only I don't think he will believe me, but now that the tests are all different, he should! Also, he says he hasn't had any heart pain since that first day... - G.P., Montreal"*

"For three weeks I had a disabling back injury from an accident, causing excruciating pain when lying down. During the healing treatment I was asleep, and when I woke up the pain was completely removed, and never returned.- F.W., Arizona"

"I wanted to have another baby, but couldn't get pregnant. I am 40 years old, and you healed me 3 months ago. I am now 2.5 months pregnant! I wanted to let you know! Thank you for God in my life again, and Joy, which is what I will name her if it's a girl! - A.M., United Kingdom"

"Dear Tiffany, healing does work! In my left ear hear sounds, loud! And the name you gave of the woman who passed away and wanted to give me love, I have received information that was my grandmother's name. And you mentioned my daughter, to take her for blood tests. In fact, she does some complain about pain inside her body. I am much calmer than before...I have been deaf since birth... Thank you! - J.O., California"

"For 18 months I suffered from an injury to my arm - hyper-extension of muscles, tendons, and almost a complete separation of the shoulder. Various therapies did little to help and the muscles were even beginning to atrophy. On Dec. 4th I had a distant healing and the results were nothing short of miraculous. The pain relief was instantaneous. Now on March 5, I can't tell

the injury ever happened. The muscles began to rebuild, the strength returned. I have no limitations - from loading wood for the heater to using my computer. God is good and Tiffany has a gift to be the conduit for those of us who need her help. If you have a doubt - DON'T - distant healing does work. Praise God and Bless Tiffany. - K.J., Alabama."

"Hello Tiffany, well, all my back pain is gone. I have had people pray over me for this debilitating pain for years. Now you pray over me once, and I am healed. I even waited two weeks to see if it would come back, and it has not. I don't understand it, unless you only choose to work on people that are about to get better, there is no logical reason for my healing. I have to say God has gifted you, and you truly are who you say you are. I am healed. I am amazed. - M.W., MD., Ohio"

First Things First

Many people confuse the terms spiritual healing with Divine healing. *Spiritual healing* can be Reiki, Therapeutic Touch,® Qigong, Quantum healing, etc. Spiritual healing may employ some sort of spiritual aspect with the healing, and may or may not include prayer. Also, the person facilitated for healing may or may not be including his own energy combined with the healing. *Divine healing* includes prayer *with* the chosen modality, cannot activate without it, and healing is never done by including any of the person's own energy. Specific prayerful intention (SPI) is what is added to Divine healing, and what we will be using with this successful method of distant healing.

Like most modalities of spiritual healing, Divine healing can be facilitated with the person in the room, or at a distance. My book *The Power of Divine: A Healer's Guide – Tapping into the Miracle* gives step by step instructions, question and answers, and numerous miraculous stories.

Like this book, find information that focuses on education and real-life experiences of healers and their methods, so that you have a "buffet" of sorts to pick and choose from to see which ones fit your palate the best. This will be an encouragement to you in your work, and the good ones can be placed on your bookshelf as reference guides for later. Remember adding prayer to the modality is what creates the miracles!

I am so pleased with the emails and letters I receive about the phenomenal healings that take place by utilizing this amazing process. There is such a need for healers, and I am very grateful to help stimulate more minds and hearts to be part of this great adventure. It is my hope that this book *Forward From the Mind* will build upon that earlier foundation, and take you beyond where you ever thought you could go, which is well beyond the basics, and into the mystical aspects of the depths of the soul.

An Honest Appraisal – Are You a Healer?

So many people ask me; *"Do you think I could be a healer?"* This is not a question that an outsider can answer - this is only for you and The Big Guy to decide. But, first we need to make our Free Will intention known, and follow through with what we need to do on our side, as if it is already accomplished. There is a "testing" of sorts that occurs, and you will be presented for opportunities to "walk your walk and talk your talk."

Many healers are called from lives that have presented them with brokenness of all sorts, with many advanced learning opportunities on a physical, emotional and spiritual level. Hence, the familiar term "wounded healer." We have had critical opportunities to choose light over darkness, love over fear, and self*less*ness over selfishness; numerous chances to choose empathy and experience fellow-feeling. That is my background too - my life has been saturated with loneliness, abuse, heart-break, poverty, overwhelming responsibility and brokenness of every kind. So how could I ever sit in judgment over anyone else, clogging up my healing channel of love for them? I have *been* everyone else! This empathy allows me to love my clients deeply and profoundly, it allows me to identify with their soul, and allow a flowing of Spirit touching spirit.

I had the choice at every dark occurrence to become hard, bitter, withdrawn, hate God and give up; or to develop empathy, forgiveness for myself and others, keep reaching out, search for God, and keep on going. *We all have the same choices.* We may not know why things are the way they are at the time,

120

but when we keep looking for the brightness, *the sun does come out,* and dry up all the rain. It is while climbing the mountain that we become strong, not the easy walking in the meadow below. And when we see the view from the top, words can't describe it to those who are still on the ground. Would I have consciously chosen the mountain trail or rock face for myself? *Heck no!* Would I now give up all the joy, miracles, adventure, multitudes of friends and true fulfillment that I experience everyday? *No way!* I am so very thankful for my life today - whatever I had to learn, whatever I needed to release to get to the bliss of where I am now, is fine with me. Everything has been leading me to the real meaning of *active and unrestrained* Unconditional Love, and the giving and receiving of it.

On this note, I want to say that I do not believe that God ever makes bad events happen in our lives. Through cause-and-effect of our own choices, environmental pollutants, genetic frailties, and dark Angelic manipulation of our Free Will, we have many different factors to contend with. But, while Divine Love never said it would be easy, He did say we would never be alone – and we have the power to align ourselves and get strong and get out of these bad situations, no matter what caused them. You do not have to be a victim here.

Healing as a journey reminds me of our car's needs - to check the fuel level, tire pressure, and cover the basics before we get too much farther down the road. It is time to ask yourself a few good questions, *that only you will be able to answer.* You are not going to get graded with a red ink pen, or have a black mark on a name chart in front of the class. You just need to make an honest appraisal of your reasons and experience in regards to this road you are on, and realize how far you've already come, and realize where the journey might lead.

Eight Questions to Ask Yourself

(1). Do you feel a real passion to heal? Does the thought of it occupy your mind constantly? Have you taken every opportunity to learn more about it, and to fully experience it yourself – in giving and receiving? The persistence, determination, and surrender needed to be tuned into the highest frequency at

the drop of a hat is a passionate and all-consuming one. You will not be afraid to offer healing at any occasion, in front of people, or at a time that is awkward for you. You are constantly looking for opportunities to try a new thing, which also embraces a child-like wonderment for healing plants, animals, the earth - in person and at a distance.

(2). Have you been reading everything you can get your hands on about healing? Do you talk to others involved in the field? Have you checked to see if the local hospitals offer various alternative medicine programs, including a recognized healing modality? Have you volunteered? Is Amazon.com your best friend? Do you have all the Internet websites on "healing" saved in your Favorites list? Do you subscribe to so many magazines and newsletters on healing that you could write one yourself? Do you write them? Do you go to all the functions you can in your area about healing, and participate in as many events as possible? Do local healers know you by name, and are you are a source of information and encouragement for them, and them for you? There is no need for judgment or competition. The proof is in the pudding - there is enough work for everyone, and the right person will be brought to the right healer. Do you believe this?

(3). How many years or how much time have you been actively involved in healing? In the music business, there is a standard joke about the 30 year old person who brags about how he started playing piano when he was only four years old. Assuming he must be a proficient player, an audition is scheduled, where he performs, at best, as an amateur. When asked why, his reply is: *"Oh, I haven't played for years – I stopped when I was 10!"* It's not the years that have gone by, it is how much you have done in the time period given you. The person with two years of experience who sees 50 different people per week has more experience than the person who sees Aunt Cleo twice a month for ten years.

(4). Do your friends and family know about your healing intentions? If you are not brave enough to let your closest friends and relatives know what is in your heart, you might have to work on some ego issues. Ego can be a lack of self-confidence, anxiety about what people will think of you, and fear of failure - ego stimulates fear. If you are fearful, you are clogging up the channel

122

for Connection, and living at a low frequency where little light can shine, and little opportunity will arise. Realize how Loved you are, how integral you are to the matrix of life and learning, and that you have the freedom to shine your light wherever you want, without any apologies to anyone. Bask in the warmth of self-confidence, and others will come to warm themselves in your fire, thankful for who you are and what you can do to help them glow as well.

(5). If you attend church, are healing services part of the program? Do you participate? If you are part of a religion that does not believe in modern day healing, you will have a difficult time staying there while advancing in this work. The secret won't stay a secret for long, as God will be utilizing you. Word will get out. This may come from people who have been healed by your hands, or may be Holy Spirit healing people around you in church, they even being "slain in the spirit" and falling down at your feet under the Power. I have been thrown out of several churches because God wanted to heal folks, but the pastors did not. Holy Spirit doesn't follow man's rules, and won't be put into time slots orchestrated to glorify men's presentations. Yet, there are many churches who do believe in healing. Find one that will support your work simply for the mutual benefit of mankind and Godly love. Some churches may already have healing rooms in place, and a group you can work with. Don't be afraid to be different in your healing approach. Each of us makes and receives Connection in his own unique, prayerful way.

(6). Are you able to get yourself out of the way and see clients as fully healed and whole? Some people who come to see you are still going to die. Some people will receive miracles. If you feel like a failure one time and a hero the next, you are giving yourself way too much credit, and way too much pressure. There are many reasons, some of which you may never know, of why one case is a cure and another is not. You are simply the conduit or power line (healer) between the electric company (Source), and the house in the neighborhood (client). It is your job to be available for *unobstructed current* to flow to the house for *any* light switch or energy needs that get switched on. You are not the one in charge. The owner of the house still has to turn on the switch. Let's take this example further:

Every house already is hard-wired to begin with, and it is up to the owner of the house to switch "on" the current to flow, and to recognize *there is a contract in place with the power company.* Since you are familiar with the usage of power and have been trained by the power company, sometimes you will also receive calls as an electrician. For this you will need to answer questions on wiring and such, so it is good for you to have studied the power company's manuals (Holy Books - scriptures). Some people in the neighborhood may want to put you on a pedestal when "all the lights come on," but they will also blame you if they don't. Just be humble, and have faith that your conduit is fine, that you know how to use the tools, and that the power company works 24/7 and you have the private service number if you have a need to call in at any time (prayer). Also recognize and appreciate that there are other electricians available to help people besides you (others called to healing).

Remember, it is always possible that a different electrician will be called in to finish the project later, or that first a homeowner will see the need to upgrade and install greater wattage bulbs (make choices of love not fear) or more lamps because their home is too dark (seeing a need for spiritual awareness), which has nothing to do with the conduit or electrician himself. Also, the power company may contact them directly (visions, dreams, etc.) or use you to relay needed information for other upgrades (word of knowledge). There are many factors to consider in this line of work, which compares favorably to the life work of a healer.

(7). Are you able to self-initiate an OOBE? To participate in this most advanced form of distant healing, this is prized. To be able to combine an out of body state with prayer is the highest form of healing I have witnessed. It makes the opportunity better for being a channel of pure healing light with fewer distractions. For example, if a healer has a cold or other health issue, the Energy is going to work first for the healer before going through to the client, and that restricts the channel. Not so if the healer has no body to channel it through.

There are other things that can cause a "cloudiness" to occur in a one-to-one healing, such as outside distractions or office noise, restriction of time, or an excess of conversation. Some people do respond better with clinical hands-on healing, because they need the touch-stone of a real person, the heat and tingling from your hands, and casual conversation to ease their minds and voice their concerns. But for those who are able to, the OOB-DH is an incredible event to participate in, a place full of miraculous interventions. If you are not able to OOBE, setting SPI and using the teddy bear as a stand-in for the client will produce good results.

(8). Have you been combining prayerful intention with your healing? Prayer is one of the most successful modalities, and one of the simplest. Anyone can send love and good thoughts and intentions to a loved one a far distance away. Prayer activates the intention to be fulfilled beyond what we could "wish" for. Nothing ever prevents us from connecting to Source, at any time, in any place. *The fact that religion has survived is proof that prayer works.* Infinitely faster than the speed of light, our compassion and prayers move at the velocity of Love. It is where the miracles happen, when you tap into Source, you go beyond anything your own energy could ever do. Also, you have "the phone on" to answer questions as you ask them, direct to Universal Mind. Without prayer, healing is like playing doctor and walking into surgery alone, without a staff or the necessary tools to help you. With prayer, you are the nurse working as an assistant to the Great Physician, and you'll see medical history in the making right over your shoulder.

Some Distant Healing Statistics

"When Jesus had entered Capernaum, a centurion came to him, asking for help. "Lord," he said, "my servant lies at home paralyzed and in terrible suffering." Jesus said to him, "I will go heal him." The centurion replied, "Lord, I do not deserve to have you come under my roof. But just say the word, and my servant will be healed...Then Jesus said to the centurion, "Go! It will be done just as you believed it would." And his servant was healed that very hour." (Mt. 8:5-13) See also Matthew 15:21-28.

According to the results back from our preliminary distant healing (DH) questionnaire, most of the clients who scheduled a healing were Caucasian females. They had over two years of college, and had tried conventional medicine before and didn't like the results they received. Most of them had moderate health problems and had tried various forms of alternative medicine and had been happy with it. Half of them had previously tried distant healing and received help, even though half of those had not yet experienced a *local* hands-on healing. Most of them believed the healing would work before they tried it, and most of them knew someone who had benefited from a distant healing. After experiencing the DH, a large percentage reported heightened states of physical, emotional, and spiritual health. Was this educated crowd satisfied enough with the results to tell others about their experience? The large percentage is exhilarating:

(67). *Would you recommend DH to others as a integrative medicine?* Yes! There are benefits from distant healing (92%) I don't know yet (5%) No, I don't think it works (3%)

Prayer is a Simple Method for Distant Healing

Prayer is *not* wishful thinking, hypnosis or mind control. It is *not* the power of positive thinking or simply encouraging the spirit within. It has consistent, measurable results. It is *not* about begging or rehearsing a set repetition of words or making trades or needing to talk anyone into anything. It is not about begging. It is simply Connection to Source, opening your mind and heart to the God of Love in the same way that you would a respected and trusted friend - with joy, humility, gratitude and thanks.

This raises your frequency beyond your self; and like a drop of dew falling into the river, you find yourself part of a Flow that leads to a mighty ocean. When you are part of this Flow, you might even feel your structure changing for the needs at hand, such as when you are in the astral state or spirit body. You may find yourself as mist, or condensation, or ice, or snow, and finally back as a drop of dew, having been a witness to everyday miracles in the process of life and death, and being a part of it all.

Such it is with the life of a healer who uses prayer. It transcends any "normal" experience, and becomes a spring of water in a parched desert. And it is important to develop your own communication pattern with the Almighty, the main point is not *how to pray,* but just *to pray!*

126

This combination of specific prayer intent (SPI) and the out-of-body state allows for tremendous ability to give and to receive. *All* information, ability and knowledge is attainable. What will you do with it? Will you believe what the eyes of the soul are telling you, or continue to look through the hazy mist that human ego and fear has enveloped you with? You will look at things differently after these empirical experiences. The question is, will you believe what you have personally learned fist-hand, or instead, only keep the handed-down information that you were taught to believe?

"...this sudden transport of the spirit, may be said to be of such a kind that the soul really has left the body...he feels as if he has been in another world, very different from this in which we live, and has been shown a fresh light there, so much unlike any to be found in this life that, if he had been imaging it, and similar things, all his life long, it would have been impossible for him to obtain any idea of them. In a single instant he is taught so many things all at once that, if he were to labour for years on end in trying to fit them all into his imagination and thought, he could not succeed with a thousandth part of them...the eyes of the soul see much more clearly than we can ordinarily see things with the eyes of the body; and some of the revelations are communicated to it without words..." Interior Castle by Teresa of Avila (16th century)

CHAPTER 9
The Full Out-of-Body Distant Healing –
A Unique Method
Where Miracles Happen; How to Activate a Healing OOBE

There are many methods for distant healing and what works for some people might not work for others. But, my favorite and *most successful method* is described here. You can adapt it as you wish. This is a very advanced method, and relies on the fact that you have a fair amount of experience already in several of these steps. With this method, you need excellent ability to shift from one level of perception to another. It is like being re-born into a higher state of being, as you shift the center of your interest from the natural to the Supernatural plane. While we are there, we become immersed in an attainment of communion, in a perfect resonance of the Oneness of all life, where anything can happen, and often does! Now let's take the process step by step:

(1). *Organize Your Tools* - Have a first and last name, year of birth, city, state and country (and photo or other trinket if possible) of the person you can hold during the distant healing. Have the identifier number available, just as you did for RV. At this time, review your previous medical intuitive notes, which you might have remote viewed only minutes before. In some cases, you might want to schedule the healing at a different time than the RV, or even the DH on its own without notes, as in successive healings. It is up to you and the client. Sometimes after I remote view, I will organize several DH before coming back to inspect new changes with RV. This saves time, and the client money.

If this DH is at a different time than the previous RV, you have confirmed the appointment time according to when the client will be asleep. In both cases, for RV or DH, during sleep is best. Remember the 10% of the brain acts as a bridge or barrier to the acceptance of healing. Being asleep helps makes a *bridge.*

(2). *Get Comfortable* - As with the process for setting up the session of medical intuition, turn off the phones, and make sure Junior and Fluffy are taken care of and out of the room. Make sure your bladder is empty. Something light in your stomach is good so you won't be brought back by hunger pains. Muted light seems more conducive than bright. Now, take one last look at the large World or United States map on the wall and see what general location you will be going to. And, if you are new to OOB and need a focal point to look at for activation, such as a rotating spiral on a laptop screen, now is the time to set it up so you can "click out" easier.

Now, find an upright comfortable chair which is tall enough to support your head, put your feet over a small ottoman (still tuck a pillow under your knees), a pillow under each arm (so your shoulders are supported), a pillow in the small of your back, and a pillow or eye sachet pillow under your chin (so your head doesn't fall forward when relaxed). I always put chapstick on my lips and around my nostrils, since if you are gone a long time, drying out can occur. If you "click out" while breathing through your mouth, you are really going to have dryness problems; a wet washcloth helps with this, but I have found much less trouble with just using the nostrils for breathing instead.

I start with an audible prayer, so the energy of the room is raised to a bright and high vibration. Then, as my relaxation progresses, I also say a quiet prayer, including an intention which prepares me for protection from any negativity, if I should meet any shadow obstacles along the way. If an assistant is there, he can read off the person's identifier number again and the basic intuitive notes/request and location, as you go deeper into relaxation. Now you can quiet your mind, focus on slowing down your heart rate and breathing, and one last time look at the picture, artifact or identifier for this person who you are connecting with. Remember your intent to stay in real-time.

(3). *Start the OOBE, Mind Awake, Body Asleep* - You are already "in synch" with the client, since you are familiar with her from the remote viewing. This makes it even easier for you to go to her now. Feel yourself sinking into the funnel and out from your body, going to the client. Or, close your eyes and rock yourself back and forth in your mind until you fall out and forward. Or,

130

see your consciousness as a small pea of white light just above your eyes, a distance out from your forehead, and gradually moving away. See yourself moving out across the room, over the distance, and exactly to the client's room, where you were before with the remote viewing.

Initiate any one of the techniques available for astral projection, and know that this is real, can be controlled by thought, is a natural state and that it happens to you every night when you sleep. The only difference is this: *mind awake!* Keep the intention strong - this is where the passion comes in - now go to the edge of consciousness, and let go even of body awareness... Out through the top of your head, or bounced straight up from your stomach, or floating up and turning over, or sitting up and rolling out - many are the doors to freedom! *Freedom!*

Everything will look much different in this out of body state than the remote viewing state. Since you are not in your body anymore, your full focus is here, and your hearing is more sensitive, light is more intense, etc. But remember, your real agenda is that you are out to heal. If you have not yet traveled to the client, intent it strongly now, and you will immediately find yourself there. Bring a full amount of Love and Peace into this room, take the same procedure that you have as an "earthly" healer and apply them here, including whatever technique you use in a clinic, you can visualize and it will occur here.

The method you use here does not make a difference to the client, what you choose is for your *own* habit or benefit, to make *you* feel comfortable. It is a "touch-stone" for your own healing reality. Sometimes I still go through the motions of placing my hands on the client, or softly rotate them in the air over the body, hold their hand, or place my hands on their head or at their feet. Now, continue to raise your vibration and intention of connection to Divine Love. My best and highest frequency to tap into are my NDE memories, and how it felt to stand in the midst of Ultimate Love and before Christ and Father. So for me, when I connect with this, it becomes a release for the outpouring of Spirit to flood the room, Spirit touching spirit, for full healing wherever it is needed.

131

At this time, you will often be witness to the client's entire body beginning to shift through different color patterns. Like a rainbow of oil on a water puddle, iridescence occurs until the colors become brilliant, and become a whitish-golden glow, like tiny shimmering stars in a Milky Way! Often there is spiraling with this glow of colors too, like looking at a cosmic event in space... it is incredible! Almost like a "new creation" occurring right then and there, in front of your very eyes. And it is hard to explain; but when you see it happening to someone else, you feel it in yourself too. It is as if you become the client for a while. Without caring and empathy for the client, this can't happen. A healer has to surrender all for each and every one, a healer has to love each person like they've never felt love before, and their cells will know it, and you will be like the rainstorm upon their parched land. But you do not become depleted, because it is not your energy, you are simply a portal of intention and focus for it. It's all about love! And without that, nothing happens.

During the session, you are there encouraging mind, body and spirit of the person to soak this all in, and opening hearts (yours and theirs - you are standing beside them in the gap) to this "super-radiance" of supreme connection, Light and Love, in gratitude and humility. As in hands-on healing, this is not something just being "done" to them, they have to willfully accept and participate too. The amount of healing they receive is not about you, except that you keep the conduit clear. See and intention them glowing, filling with Spirit, luminescent!

You may see the darkness of the injured places that you intuitively saw in RV, and often you will see them change, and even disappear as all this is occurring. Even when you do see these places melt away, you *must not diagnose this* unless you are also a medical doctor, and the client must stay on any medications until his doctor tells them otherwise. Your job will be to encourage the person to get *new* tests done, and the healing will be verified by this. After the glow starts to go down, you can decide to come back to your home body, or go play! Since you had an identifier to get here, that has allowed you a "passport" which held a space for you in a particular place. It would be hard for me to just go to Austria, for example, on my own. But, on invitation and with an "area code," I have a touch-stone, a road-map of a sort.

132

It allows me to get there. So, most of the time I go play for a bit, but sometimes you are not quite done yet…

(4) Bilocation? - Always check for this! Much information and details about this extraordinary adventure can be found in a later chapter. Most of the time you will know when bilocation (BL) is occurring, because you can feel something different is happening, and the power through you changes as you solidify. If this is the case, the person will always wake up, because there is a purpose for it, *and you will not go unseen.* Most of the time, bilocation will *not* happen, but only a manifestation, mist or apparition appears of you. Other times, partial manifestation occurs, and features are quite clear. In both cases you can talk and often be heard. With a full manifestation you can also be touched and felt. One of the most common aspects of BL is when just my hands, face or arms appear. It is a strange feeling to have a body-part manifestation, it's similar to when a limb "goes to sleep" and imaginary ants move up it. It definitely feels different than a full body BL, the electrical charges are different, and more pronounced than the places that do not form. You will just have to experience it. When this happens, the body parts still feel different for quite a while after you return to your home body. I don't know why this is the case. The chapter on BL will fill you in on more specifics.

When You BL, You Attract Others Who BL Too

Like attracts like, and if you have a high energy and good connection with Source, then you find yourself as a team player - and others will be brought to you who *also bilocate.* Some of them you may never see in any other way! All of this is Divine Intervention and will help you, and they, accomplish their purpose. Some will be further along in their journey than you are, and you can learn from them. Others will learn from you. I find there are always new things to learn from one another, no matter what we are working on at the time.

You will always be able to recognize these souls of enlightenment after you feel the difference of yourself in a manifested body compared to your physical body. And, emotionally, these team players are a light to the world. They exude gentleness, peace, purpose, and high inspiration. They know they are a candle in the dark, and do not fear the shadow, nor feel a need to compete.

They are living the great life, and always in a state of junction and connection between mind and matter - between the candle and the flame. Almost like the quark itself, which flickers in and out of space (while physicists ponder where it goes), life pulsates within them. Remember, you will attract the wave lengths that oscillate at your frequency. If you are attracting illness and negativity that will also be reflected in the people around you, like to like. You need to ask yourself where changes should occur, and the opportunity for change will appear in front of you. Repeatedly so - until the change is made! And you will attract and illuminate brightness.

"When you are around them (connector people), you feel energized, purposeful, inspired, and unified. You're seeing people whom you want to hang around with because they energize you, and this brings you a feeling of empowerment. When you feel empowered and energized, you step into the flow of abundant Source energy yourself, and you inadvertently invite others to do the same. The connection isn't just to Source energy, it's to everyone else and everything in the universe. Connectors are aligned with the entire cosmos and every particle within the cosmos. This connection makes the infinite power of intention possible and available." – The Power of Intention by Dr. Wayne Dyer

Sometimes you will make friends in the astral out of body world, who are other folk traveling in astral form. You only meet them while *you too* are out of body (unless you are sensitive and can see other dimensions) and they are easy to recognize as travelers instead of bilocaters. This has been very interesting for me, since all this is empirical information, and there is such little information on it. But it makes sense in the big picture. Since The Big Guy coordinates all this, wouldn't He bring people together for answers, to befriend one another, or to help with a group project? All of us are linked together in this field of opportunity, intention and interaction with one another and Him. Here is an experience of that, that healing can be beyond helping just the physical body.

Group Project: Out-of-Body Experience on 9-11

On the evening of September 11th 2001, the day of the desolation of the Twin Towers, I felt a definite "calling" to make myself available for the astral work, which I did. Lying on top of a stone picnic table on a cliff overlooking the sea, with two of my best friends with me, I prayed, reached out my mind…and disappeared out of body. Although this is a long story, I hope it is one that will encourage you to astral travel, and to see another avenue that you can help others with your out of body experiences (excerpted from my book *Psychic Gifts in the Christian Life - Tools to Connect*).

"…From above I saw my body on the table and my companions all around me. I knew my body would be safe. I saw the twilight of dusk glowing orange over the sea. Then I felt my consciousness go straight up into the sky; so high that I could not even see where the ocean met the shore. I was out of my body, but I was not afraid. From my consciousness in the sky, I saw rapid movement of clouds and light around me, although it was getting dark, and a blur of speed, and then felt a feather lightness of descending toward the ground. I had traveled a great distance in a very short period of time….In front of me, hanging in the air at varying heights, were translucent white objects, thousands of them glowing, each one being six to seven feet high and about three feet wide. As I got closer, I saw definition in the midst of the radiant glowing. I saw faces. These objects were scores of ghostly white spirits - they were hanging in mid-sky above a destruction of debris. I had been brought to the twin towers, in New York City…

I saw immensely bright Angels (tall, about 9 feet high) placed here and there, and they were helping the people who had died. There were other spirits with the Angels, these had a bluish-white color, they seemed to be the friends and family of those who had died. They were there to help the transition. There was no hurry. Every now and then I would see an Angel going upward, the new spirit in tow, with the odd bluish-white spirits behind, pulling up the rear in a semi-circle. There was a subtle white "funnel" over the top of this area, which I guessed was used as a transportation device to where they needed to go…and evidently, this had to have been going on all day…

Also to the side of me there floated an Angel; and there were two other spirits near him. He motioned me to come over, and instantly I was there. A woman

135

in a spirit body introduced herself to me as (sounds like) "Asa'ri-ta." I had the feeling that she was an astral traveler who had been sent for, just like me. She glowed differently than the friends and family - there were many of us called here in our astral bodies, which were still living on earth, we were the ones glowing blue...

The next thing I knew, I was in one of the planes! I was beside a child of 4 or 5 years of age - her mother was on the other side, and didn't seem to know I was there. We could see the tower in front of us; the plane was heading straight into it. I felt terror in my heart - so much fear, and confusion! I was re-living and relieving the last few moments of this child's life. I was sharing her emotion; it was if she and I were the same. Her emotions clinging to me, our minds as one. Her knowing she was not alone. The fear escalated within us - I looked past the girl and saw her mother, round eyes in silent shock facing forward. I see other passengers, shrieking and screaming and climbing over the seats, falling over each other.

I see the terrorists; two men with dark skin, one way up by the open cockpit door, the other to the left in front of the passengers. They are shouting loudly in a foreign tongue over the screams. It seemed by the faces and the shouts of the one beside the cockpit door, that he was shouting with joy. The other one was screaming in fear. I felt my stomach turn over.

We hit. I feel the release of letting go...there is no pain! The worst part is the fear beforehand. I have died with the girl. There is no pain from the death. Now she has relived it, and I am standing here in front of her, her glow just one of the thousands around me. Evidently, this "re-living" had been going on all day. It was time for the cycle of fear to stop. It was time for her to go Home.

I look in her beautiful eyes, face to face. I tell her it is OK, and not to be afraid. I tell her that she is Loved by God, and that her family is waiting for her. I think all these things in my mind, and know that she can hear me, telepathically. I remember my own experiences of going before the Presence - the feeling of all-encompassing love. I project the experience to her in my mind. She smiles. She understands. She wants to go home. I feel the pang of

136

wanting to go home too, to Father. I look above and see the relatives - five or six bright faces, some with their arms open toward her. She turns back to me and I hear her question in my head, "where's mom?"

I am back in the airplane. Now I am sitting where the girl used to be, alongside the mother who is in shock. I see the passengers; I look around and notice even more than I did before. I see the terrorists. I hear their words again. One is younger than the other, and is in a brother-like relationship - submissive to the other. The dominant one has a symbol on his upper right shoulder - somehow I can see it under his jacket.

Again I feel the growing terror. The fear mounts. It is overwhelming; we feel that we will burst from fear. We hit...again, there is no pain. We are floating. We have been released. The woman's glow is before me, I tell her it is O.K., and not to be afraid. She looks me in the eyes. I recall to her my near-death experiences of heaven. I tell her that her child is safe and is among the relatives waiting to greet her. I tell her she can go to the Light of God, now, or stay until the funeral is over, but suggested she leave now. I tell her she will be allowed to visit here on earth later, if she so wishes.

An Angel comes to our group, and descends gently amongst us. The brightness is beyond "white." Angels have such a high vibration! It is much easier to see the details of them with my existing in a spirit form, as compared to wearing my fleshly body. In my physical body, it is hard to make out facial features of Angels, everything is bleached out with brightness. There is a whirring sound, like a vibration, that corresponds with the presence of these Angels. I look intently, wanting to memorize every detail, this experience is so extraordinary.

For the first time, here I see that wings are actually shafts of energy radiating out from their bodies! The Angel starts to ascend, with his entourage of mother and child, and supportive relatives and friends. My body feels like lead weight. I want to go too! Let me go too!!! Their group glow gets absorbed by the funnel of light. I can't see them anymore. I feel sad for myself, but happy too. It is like the feeling of a mother at the graduation of her child, knowing the young adult needs to move on without her.

137

Next, I help a young blonde pregnant woman (she is only 2-3 months along); a woman in her 50's; and one of the pilots, who met with a violent death before crashing into the tower. Five people. Five deaths. Each time I had to relive (and relieve), the last few moments of their lives, when the fear was so great (especially for the 50's woman, who had not believed in God all her life and was really fearful of death), and then the blissful release.

I saw the final moments so clearly that I knew where people were sitting, and felt I could even draw a diagram and sketch their faces. I especially paid attention to the details of the terrorists. It was like a movie repeating over and over again.

The main terrorist, who killed the pilot, also was the leader of this group. He is the one with the symbol. This man used a thin (green?) instrument to cut marks into the front wall by the cockpit; and there seemed to be foam, or a white background, seen under the cuts. At first when I saw this, I thought he was just being destructive. But, when I did a sketch of the angles of the lines, I saw what was probably the lettering of a word. He was taller than the other man by about two inches, though both were slender. I heard the sounds of the names, especially since the younger one was calling so much to the older one. The younger one was frightened. He wanted to live. He had not been shouting with joy. They were wearing headbands.

I saw many empty chairs in the front of the plane. I do not know if there were more people crowded in the back. I do not remember looking behind me, only to the front and sides. I will not relate to you the cutting of the pilot, but please know that there was not any feeling of pain with his release. I do know that his essence chose to stay for his funeral. I don't remember the choices of the others. I know the mom and daughter left together with the Angel. I had encouraged the mother to go, now. I wanted the Unconditional Love of the Father to envelope the little girl as soon as possible.

I do not know what happened to the 50's woman. The last time I saw her, she had an Angel in serious conversation with her, then I felt a draw (like a magnetic pull) and "pop!" I was immediately back in my body. No feeling of

138

travel this time, just "pop!" I remember lying on the cold picnic table, looking up at the stars. I saw I had been escorted back; just at the top of my vision I saw the familiar glow of an Angel spirit, now ascending out of sight. I felt such a peacefulness as a child of God. I praised Father for using me in such a special way. The clock said I had been gone about 40 minutes.

It was related to me by my companions that my body had tensed up and spasmed five times while I was gone. Then it would relax completely. My friends had become fearful and placed their hands on my head and feet. They had also felt and seen a definite jolt when I "popped" back in. Under the pin-lights of the stars, in the cool sea breezes blowing up the bluff, I related to them my experiences. We all cried. We prayed. And we praised The Great Comforter.

The FBI - "Let Us Know…We Keep a File"

Two days later I jotted down the phone number that had been advertised on TV for contacting the FBI with any information on the terrorists. I had hoped for a fax machine number, since I had also made sketches of the tattoo, the slashes/word on the wall, and the face of the main terrorist. These could not be explained, but had to be shown. I called the number and asked the man I was talking to if they had a fax machine. He said "No. We don't have one." He asked what I had, and how I got it. After skirting around about "how I got it," I went on to tell him what I had. Half way through he stopped me and said: "Here's our fax number." I asked him, "Whom do I direct it to?" He said "No one; I am going to go stand by it and wait." I smiled to myself.

Evidently God had given me some information that they already knew - enough that this fellow knew that this was not rubbish, and to question if it might contain other accurate information too. Maybe something there helped on the investigation. At this early time the press had released very little to the public. The FBI was keeping information close to them, guarding things well.

He continued, "Let us know whenever you work with the police departments…we keep a small file on hand. There is a small group we run things by at times. The FBI is not closed to unusual methods of retrieval (of

139

information). There is also some money involved." I swallowed hard. I couldn't believe this guy was being so open with me. Here was proof that the FBI does use "sensitives" in their work! Evidently I had some information that corresponded accurately with something they knew, that had not been released yet. It seemed he was convinced that I could "qualify" for this group at some time.

As the days went on, I watched the news more and more. Terrorist names and faces appeared, including the two I knew. They announced headbands - red ones, and other points of validation through time...it was all familiar to me...but the real gift had been the honor to be called there by The Big Guy to help release fear, and transition them to the ocean of Love awaiting them..."

So as you can see, the OOB can be a "group effort" experience, and useful for many kinds of healing, even unto death and transition. In this case, from a ghost-like state into the freedom of the spirit, unencumbered by physical perceptions and helped by Angels and those still alive but out working while in the astral body.

Do Weather Conditions, Diets, Drugs, Holidays, Alter Distant Healing?

I see this question primarily targeted to the OOB healing event itself, and secondly to the RV. There are several opinions; and I will add my own, but your own experience should be your ultimate answer. Since sensory abilities encompass a wide range, I am including here research on other modalities as well.

"The entire body of dream research data from Maimonides Medical Center, selecting the first night that each subject in a telepathy experiment had visited the laboratory. They matched the results of these nights with geomagnetic data, discovering that the subjects' telepathy "hits" tended to be higher during calm nights than during nights marked by electrical storms and high sunspot activity..." - Persinger & Krippner, 1989.

Personal habits influence us in our normal, day-to-day life. Why should we think any differently about how our habits influence our RV and OOB time?

140

Some things can actually prevent success in attaining "the zone," and suppress your ability to control the processing of information in your mind. Other things stimulate the nervous system, and will make it harder to quiet the noise and clear the mental screen. Not sleeping enough, being sick, over-worked and exhausted, all these things will have a negative impact. Take care of yourself! Your body is the vehicle to catapult you beyond it - so respect and value it!

"We propose two interpretations of the geomagnetic field effect. The first is that psi is a geomagnetic field correlate; solar disturbances and consequent geomagnetic storms affect this correlate. The second is that the geomagnetic field affects brain receptivity to psi, which remains constant. Deep temporal lobe activity exists in equilibrium with the global geomagnetic condition. When there is a sudden decrease in geomagnetic activity, there appears to be an enhancement of processes that facilitate psi reception, especially telepathy and clairvoyance." - Persinger & Krippner, 1989.

- *Drugs & Alcohol:* Drugs are out. There is a need for control with DH. In the RV state of medical intuition, your perceptions of colors will be altered. You will not be able to process information well that you receive on any other levels, because it will be cloudy. Drugs and alcohol can put you to sleep or heighten your state of arousal. Both have an adverse effect on DH. Transferring to an OOBE state takes control and focus, and intentional release and relaxation. Some people also get paranoid when involved with chemicals. All these things lower the body's vibrations, and may entice an attack of lower form while you are in a weakened state. It is quite likely that over-the-counter medications may have some adverse effects on these modalities too; *when in doubt, don't go "out."*

- *Weather Conditions:* I have *not* found snow, rain, sun nor any other weather condition to negatively affect DH. I *have* found the temperature of the room or the bed to be a factor, you should be warm, but not hot, or else a panic sets in and your body will call you back from your travels prematurely. Humidity does seem to help, and the nasal passages like it too. Also, if you have a personal fear of lightning or thunder, then this will subconsciously depress your ability to be successful. For me, since my NDE I feel drawn to it and

141

really enjoy "clicking out" when the environmental energy is so effervescent and high. If you go out at night, or to somewhere that is dark, saying *"clarity now"* or *"brightness now"* should help any murkiness. I find the colors are a bit more muted, and they look orangey to me. For new OOBErs, the ability to see all around you instead of just in front where your eyes normally are is probably the hardest thing to get used to. There is little perception of what is up or down, right or left; which is why ghosts seem to be "floating" back and forth, they are struggling with it too. It gets a bit easier with time, just be patient.

- *Diet:* This is probably one of the most disputed subjects. Some people say fasting helps. I have regularly fasted for about a month or so each year, and I have seen a correlation of a "loosening" effect beneficial for DH after about the 14th day, and again around the 21$^{st.}$ As a side note, fasting does not help RV, where an active consciousness is needed to retain focus. On the opposite side, eating a heavy meal beforehand will put you to sleep; since all the body's energy would be concentrated there, with nothing left to support pure-energetic activity. Afterward you come back from your excursion, eating something light and drinking water will help "ground" you back into your body. Many healers eat no red meat (I am one of these), and consume only organic vegetables and fish or make other careful food regime choices. Not one of these things is absolute. It is useful to recognize *your* body and soul's own choices, and be true to them, not what someone else tells you. A highly trained intuition and connection to one's self and Spirit will tell you all you need to know.

- *Body Position:* Most people seem to feel this doesn't matter. To me, it definitely does. I have found it easier to be head-first in a North-to-South position. I have found it more conducive to be sitting in a chair than lying down, which can put me to sleep. When I have "clicked out" lying down, it has been easier to be on my back, facing up - face down was impossible, and going "out" while lying on my side was difficult and only accomplished with the "rolling" technique. Generally I leave through the top of my head; perhaps that has something to do with my personal choice of body position. I have found gentle quietness to be an aid, or just the sounds of nature as a background, and phones and such should be turned off. But, I feel that everyone should learn how to practice his modality in a less-than-perfect state. Achieving complete quietness is going to be impossible most of the time. Practice relaxation techniques and these modalities with small distractions, and you will have a better chance of success in the long-range plan, and be able to "click out" almost anywhere.

- *Sun and Moon:* Our bodies are 70% water and highly affected by gravity. This is the same as the 70% body of water on our earth, which is clearly affected by the moon in the tides. But, the astral body has no mass, so how could gravity affect it? I have not personally noticed any reactions, positive or negative, to solar flares, eclipses or new and full moons in my astral body.

- *Holidays & World Events:* I have had negative experiences and high distraction levels when working on holidays. I have certainly seen the difference, and had to scuttle and rearrange healing schedules all the time until I figured this out. The holidays of New Year, Independence Day, Halloween and at least three days leading up to Christmas have all had negative results. Why would this be so? Here is my explanation: unconscious group stress and emotions - again the mechanics of this cosmic energy soup we are living in - we feel what everyone else feels. When people are nervous, stressed about relatives and traveling, money, being alone, etc, there is a low-energy attached to it (as in the days leading up to Christmas) that wants to saturate with depression, and can lower our ability to move freely. I have noticed that this limitation has lessened over time, and as I have become brighter and am moving to a higher vibrational level, there is less notice of the lower vibrations around me.

So keep in mind that this amount of human chaos, expectation, drunkenness, loneliness and anxiety gives an additional dusting of energy that brings shadow to the forefront. It can also be harder to focus through this shattered energy fog - it can feel like a band of negative energy so close to the ground that you are literally trapped there. In "Star Wars" terms, it is a "disruption in the Force!" Whereas RV might be possible, I have found going OOB at such a time can lead to a time of vulnerability, almost like putting blood in the water for sharks. Later, we will talk about what these sharks are and protection against them. So, why not just wait for another day to go astral?

You can spend those low-energy days in an effort to raise the frequency level by prayer and love; I do the same after traumatic world events, which certainly affects people everywhere whether they know about it or not. Have you ever noticed how terrible earthquakes, Tsunamis, droughts, fires, etc. follow the highly charged emotional events of humans? It causes an imbalance in the system that affects the entire world. Is it any wonder that the highly realized *love* of Jesus could *calm* a storm? (Mt. 8:23-27) We have that power too, to damage or to mend - on a global scale, and with weather conditions. Remember the shaman's rain dances? Perhaps there was more wisdom there than we give him credit for.

Sending Healing to the Future

With distant healing, the world is your oyster! Anytime that you wish to, you can be a vessel of light and hope, even to a future event. Here is a variation of using specific prayerful intention to manifest or "store up" for a purpose and time outlined. You can even use our friendly teddy bear to be the stand-in for intention, including touching where you will want the healing done.

- *My Future Dentist Appointment:* I had an appointment to get out my old silver fillings and have them replaced with new porcelain ones. I knew what day the appointment was, and approximately what hour. Having spent years of my childhood in braces and also having had bad reactions with Novocain before, I sent DH to the date. Since I had not been at this office previously, I had nothing to visualize on except how I perceived myself with a new smile. The day came, and as I sat down in the chair and the dental assistant prepared the swab and needle for the Novocain, I asked if I could have five minutes alone first, "just some quiet time to relax." With a strange look on her face, she briefly left the room, whereby I perceived the Connection, and felt a wave of familiar warmth wash over me. I gave a silent prayer of thanks, knowing my jaw wouldn't feel like it would be dragging on the floor for five hours.

When the assistant came back in, I told her I wouldn't need any Novocain, and to proceed with the drilling. This prompted an outcry of disbelief, and the dentist was called in, to whom I had to promise that if I felt any pain, I would

144

surely let him know to stop. Four molars, including two on top, were soon successfully drilled, scraped, and replaced with new fillings. One of the top back molars was also cracked, and I received a crown on that one. The dentist would often stop as he was drilling, grinding and shaping, and ask in amazement how I was doing, to which I would give a thumbs up, or shake my head, with a sparkle in my eyes. I felt the deep pressure of the drill, and the whirling sound was disconcerting, as were the flakes flying around from the process. But I felt little discomfort, and never the need for Novocain! It was the first time the office had ever had a patient behave like this - which meant all the assistants had to come in to look. When I had a chance to tell why I didn't need it, it was with a clear voice and no effects from the procedure that I shared the secret of distant healing and prayer. Then *their jaws* dropped to the floor, and all I could do was flash my new smile, just as I had visualized it to be weeks earlier.

Sending Healing to the Past – Preventative Health

One of the most interesting parts of quantum mechanics is that the outcome isn't known until it is looked at. Then, as we have seen, it gets "locked in" to being a wave or a particle. Very interesting events have taken place with random-number-generators (RNGs) about this - a normal split of 50/50 is to be expected by a machine taping 1s and 0s, which is what you will get when you normally process the tape. But, if a tape *hasn't been looked at yet,* a person can affect change on an already recorded tape! Many times I have sent healing to the past with success. Can you see the possibilities for this? What an intervention tool - there are no end to the possibilities.

"Helmet Schmidt at the Mind Science Foundation in San Antonio, Texas, had already shown through years of work that a person could mentally interact with the machine (RNG) at a distance, to obtain more 1s or 0s just by paying attention to the desired outcome...in his latest and most remarkable experiments, he has shown that even after the machine is run and has generated a tape recording of its output of 1s and 0s, a person can still affect the outcome by paying attention to the tape, as long as no one has seen the data beforehand...We do not believe that the person is actually changing the tape, which may be a punched-hole paper tape, but rather, Schmidt and

others believe that the person with the tape in his hand is reaching back in time to affect the machine at the time of its operation...Schmidt has even demonstrated that the prerecorded, but unobserved, breathing rate of a person in the past can be affected by the mental activity of a person at a later time! Both of these experiments suggest that a healer can similarly reach back in time far enough to affect her patient's – or even her own – physiology at a point early enough where it can still do some good, and achieve a healing outcome..." -Miracles of Mind by Russell Targ and Jane Katra Ph.D.

"If these nonlocal intentions are aligned with aims or goals of health and wholeness, perhaps active intentions could be directed in the present or even into the past to promote biological and psychological seed moments favorable to physical and psychological health and well-being...If such a process could act early and thoroughly enough, it might actually prevent the development of harmful physical or psychological processes. This would constitute an instance of true preventive medicine. Time-displaced healing modalities might actually have important advantages over real-time healing modalities...consider - a small group of cancerous cells or precancerous cells at a certain location within the body and a natural killer (NK) cell that is roaming near those cells in a random or freely variable course. It is conceivable that there exists a point at which a random "choice" or "decision" occurs, and the NK cells could move, with 50/50 probability, either toward or away from those cancerous cells...in principle, intentional influences could bias the probabilities of action...thereby terminating a seed moment that otherwise might have eventuated in illness or even death." - Distant Mental Influence by William Braud, Ph.D

Finding laboratory results for "retrohealing" may be very difficult. But, I have seen positive changes in people that can be explained *very well* within this paradigm. So many times I have seen and felt, through medical intuition, *very real past problems that became current diseases.* Now, perhaps it is also through faith that I do not "set" as absolute the things I see, but I know all things can change for good. I don't conduct blood tests, or conduct any intrusive or medical procedure. Often these things are "set" by the client's doctors before they come. But is it possible that cancerous tumors, heart

146

conditions, diabetes, immune diseases, etc., might change their course by healing intention, partially because they are not yet "observed?" Remember that with prayer you work hand-in-hand with the Great Observer, and you have your answer. All things can change, no matter what got them bad to begin with.

The Invisible Miracles

In my work, I can chart the results of this by seeing the client a second time, and noting changes that have taken place by another medical intuitive scan. In positive cases, the client will also be collaborating the new facts - she'll feel better, have more energy, be sleeping soundly, have less pain, anxiety, etc. This is another reason why a person facilitated for healing cannot have need for external gratification - the point to healing is helping the client be sound and whole again, not having your ego and doubt stroked by needing everything validated and diagnosed.

I would like to point out a couple of other facts with regard to this: I find that the most well-versed clients, who know every in and out about their diagnosed malady, *are the ones hardest to heal.* The analytical brain seems to hold every statistic very close to home. These people usually try to educate me on every detail of what they have, what they've done…a step-by-step drama that *needs to be shut down very early.* For one thing, you can feel the vibration in the room lower as the client is describing all this trauma and pain, and I can feel my own frequency starting to come down too.

If the client is left to go on and on, or refuses to stop talking about it, the healing will not be a good one. You must shift this into a positive conversation, or have no conversation at all! The same for a distant healing, some folks will want to send you all the information in their files beforehand, a record of every stat and medical definition of their problem. This is not needed, just let it go!

Fear is another reason to stop analyzing the situation. The more you concentrate on the lion, the bigger and more ferocious the lion seems to be,

147

and your fear will neglect to see that the lion is paying no attention to you, and gazing only upon the gazelle by the river bank. In your fear, you probably haven't noticed the beauty of the waving gold tundra grasses and the tall white ibis in the tree, but have already envisioned yourself attacked, and pulled apart, and eaten by a predator. Now that we know how quantum mechanics works, and God and our intention in with it, that you attract what you send (or, "get what you ask for"), shouldn't you watch every thought that comes into your head? Manifest good choices for yourself, and others!

When the client voices a negative, *that lion gets bigger in my mind too!* That is why it is only necessary to tell me simple information, or none at all. And this is why, at large group healing events where I may have only 30 seconds or less with each person, we let everyone know that *"Holy Spirit is like aspirin, it goes where it's needed!"* And I heal all the wheelchair bound people and obvious ailments very soon in the program - that way I do not subconsciously give my brain an option to start a stagnating and negative dialog. This might go like this: *"You can't heal that! Don't you see how crippled he is? Don't you see the deformity of her face? These problems are too big for you? Who do you think you are? You can't help these people! Look at that body cast!"* And on and on…but why should I let myself get in the way of God and this person working together? The Creator of all things certainly knows how things work, including the human body. There is no problem too big for him. Remember, we are simply the extension cord between two points, a touchstone of unimpeded love. Why clog up the channel with our own stuff?

One more point - I have had very good healing responses also from sending healing into the past. Divorces, medical emergencies, high stress times, sexual abuse, grief - the sting becomes less when we simply pin-point a time or problem, and send love back to it. In these cases, when the client actively acknowledges the problem and allows forgiveness of the situation, the people involved, and themselves, beautiful healing occurs (see my book *"The Power of Divine: A Healer's Guide - Tapping into the Miracle"* for more information on this).

Emotional healing is another place where Supernatural intervenes and affects changes in our life and attitude that *we cannot do on our own.* I know - I have had many, many times of brokenness in my life; and the resentment, mistrust and anger was like a war waging inside of me that I needed to always be in control of. Now, I can look back on all of these situations with forgiveness of myself and others, and as just something I moved through, without any of the accompanying high emotions. It is almost like I am seeing it as another person, and truly, I have become one - peaceful and calm, and overflowing with blissfulness and love for all others, freely and without mistrust or fear. I could not do this on my own. I tried. Prayer in combination with the healing intention is needed. Free Will aligning ourselves to Loving Source dissolves the feelings of anger and separation.

Have *Fun* with Out of Body too!

It is important for us as healers to find balance in all things, and to enjoy our work! This includes taking time to explore real-time in the astral body, and also have fun in the dimensions. For fun OOB time at home, I have an over-sized "bean bag" where I can lie down, and prop it how I need it. This is much better than working on a bed where I am already programmed to go to sleep. I *only* use this place for OOB, which has helped subconsciously train my mind to quickly relax as soon as I lie down. In my play time, I usually go out in "real-time," since most of the information I wish to know about and places of interest to me are here on this plane. Sometimes I think astral travel is very similar to being a specter in this world, a living spirit moving between the dimensions, interacting invisibly and bringing back information with which to further ponder.

Since the bean bag is portable, this is also handy for putting near the window, or next to a computer to use a voice activated software program if I want to remote view something on my own. In this way, theoretically I could dictate the notes directly instead of having someone write down the information, but for me this rarely works. In real life, tape recording and electronics do not work well around me, especially in an altered or healing state, and are unreliable, stopping or only producing white noise. In any case, I also enjoy the companionship and energy of having a "live person" in the room with me, for both healing and remote viewing sessions. Now, what have the *results* been with clients with this method of remote viewing for medical intuition and out of body for distant healing?

CHAPTER 10

The Distant Healing Research Questionnaire
Nonlocality & Statistics of a Preliminary Personal Study

Does sex, age, culture or country the client lives in make a difference with the ability to benefit from distant healing? Do alcohol or prescription drugs, non-prescription drugs (such as cold or allergy medications), alcohol, sedatives or stimulants (such as coffee and tea) make a difference in bodily receptiveness? Does the client's religion, spiritual path, or lack of one play a role? Does a distant healing change the emotional or spiritual habits of a person? What is the average person's belief about what a healing is and why a healing does or doesn't occur? What percentages of clients receive immediate, spontaneous healings compared to in-process healing? Did clients know when the healing was going on, did this make a difference? How many actually received healing? How accurate is physical and emotional medical intuition for DH? Overall, what are the most beneficial results from a DH?

The distant healing research questionnaire is where I really started noticing the differences of the techniques and intentions for distant healing, medical intuition, and remote viewing. It has helped me answer all the questions above, and it has helped me to become better at the ability to perceive, receive, and give accurate interpretation of information. I am presenting the full distant healing questionnaire below that was given out to clients after the healing, so you as the reader can see the entire process from beginning to end, and understand the answers received. There was no money or compensation of any kind exchanged for filling out the questionnaire, only for the initial cost of the healing session. Most of the time, the results came back without me knowing who the person was, since by request only initials of the clients were used.

Please note that this is not a scientific or double-blind study, but according to Dr. Bruce Greyson, who was kind enough to review this questionnaire and results, this *can* be called a preliminary study. All the healings were performed only by me, and only through my own methods of Divine Healing, which in most cases includes the person being asleep while it occurs. For the skeptic, it could be that the statistics are quite high about the benefits of DH because only those who benefited from it returned the questionnaire. Also, some people desired to know the night and time of the healing, while others did not, so that might make a difference as to expectation. The information is simply offered as interesting "food for thought" from 216 willing participants. The questionnaire was sent out anywhere from immediately after the DH (with a note asking the client to wait for a week or more before completing it), to several months after (to offer the questionnaire to previous clients when the form wasn't available). Most are of the former, the newer clients.

If you find this questionnaire useful in whole or in part, *you are welcome to use as is or to adapt it to your own healing or RV medical intuitive work,* to find out the delicate nuances of what is working for you and what is not. To reduce space, all empty lines in the original questionnaire have been removed from this text. But in the original, I felt it was important for the client to be able to add additional information or thoughts about the question, and almost every question had the space for further details. There was also availability to write their entire experience in full detail at the end.

DISTANT HEALING RESEARCH QUESTIONNAIRE

Hello From Tiffany Snow! *It has been suggested that I gather and publish findings from the numerous remote healings conducted every year into book form to analyze and develop statistics to validate this method of integrative medicine. So, if you desire to share your experience and help us show the results in this field of healing, please answer the 70 questions below and mail to us at the address given, or email it.* *Thank You for Participating!*

This is a questionnaire about Distant Healing. Some of the questions may not apply to your experience. Do not be concerned about that. Just skip those questions. In many places we ask you to be specific, because details are important. However, if you do not remember some item of information exactly, write whatever you do remember. *Your name will be kept confidential, and only your first and last initials will be used for data entry and story purposes.* (Use additional pages as necessary) Distant Healing will be condensed to "DH" for the purpose of this questionnaire.

BACKGROUND

(1).   Initials of First and Last Name:
(2).   Today's Date:
(3).   Year of Birth:
(4).   Male / Female
(5).   State of Birth:
(6).   Country of Birth:
(7).   Martial Status at time of Healing: Single / Married / Divorced / Widowed / Other:
(8).   Race: Caucasian / Hispanic / Native American / Asian / African-American / Other:
(9).   Highest level of education completed:
(10).   Occupation:
(11).   What was your age at time of DH?
(12).   Month and Year of DH:
(13).   What state and country did your DH occur in?

HEALTH QUESTIONS

(14).   How would you describe your <u>physical</u> health just prior to your experience?
         Excellent Health
         Moderately Good Health, No Serious Problems
         Experienced a Serious Health Problem within 1 year before the DH
         Seriously ill at the time of the DH

(15).   Has your condition been diagnosed by a medical doctor? If so, what was the diagnosis?
(16).   Any other <u>physical</u> problems? List here:
(17).   How long have you had these problems? How did they begin?
(18).   Any family history of illness? If so, what?
(19).   Please indicate if you took any of the following substances within 48 hours prior to DH: Alcohol (type wine / beer / hard alcohol and

153

amount):

Hallucinogenic drugs (type and dose):

Prescription drugs (type and dose):

Non-prescription drugs such as cold or allergy medications (type and dose):

Pain-killers: (type and dose):

Sedatives or tranquilizers (type and dose):

Stimulants (such as coffee and tea) (type and amount):

Other: (please specify type and dose):

(20). Do you smoke? Yes / No How many packs per day?

(21). Do you exercise? How often and what kind?

(22). How would you describe your <u>mental</u> health just prior to your experience?

Excellent Emotional Health

Moderately Good Emotional Health, No Serious Problems

Experienced a Serious Emotional Problem within 1 year before the DH

Seriously ill at the time of the DH

(23). Have you been diagnosed by a mental health professional? If so, what was the diagnosis?

(24). Any family history of mental illness? If so, what?

(25). Any other emotional difficulties at time of DH? (relationship / financial / stress, etc.)

(26). How long have you had these problems? How did they begin?

(27). How would you describe your <u>spiritual</u> health just prior to your experience?

Excellent Spiritual Health

Moderately Good Spiritual Health

No interest in spiritual health

Other:

(28). What religion / spiritual path were you raised with? Denomination?

Protestant

Catholic

Jewish

Islamic

Eastern (Hindu, Buddhist)

154

Agnostic

Atheist

Other (please specify):

(29).   What religion / spiritual path are you on now?
(if none, please state that also and why)

(30).   Prior to your DH, how often were you attending religious / spiritual services?

more than once a week

once a week

once a month

occasionally or irregularly

holidays only

never

(31).   After your DH, how often are you attending religious / spiritual services?

more than once a week

once a week

once a month

occasionally or irregularly

holidays only

never

(32).   Prior to your DH, did you routinely spend time doing any of the following?

Prayer (how often?)

Meditation (how often?)

Exercise (stretching, Yoga, etc. what and how often?)

Reading or advancing knowledge (how often?)

Communion with nature (how often?)

Other (how often?)

(33).   After your DH, have any of these habits changed? Which ones and why?

(34).   Did you communicate with the healer what complaints you were asking healing for? If so, please list in detail what your requests were: (physically, emotionally, spiritually)

(35).   Were you under any unusual stress, or undergoing significant life changes, at the time of your DH?

(36).   What conventional medicine or surgery have you tried before?
        Did that help?

(37).   Are you on a special diet or way of nutrition? Also list any
        supplements here:

(38).   What alternative or integrative medicines or therapies have you
        tried before. Did that help?

(39).   Have you ever tried in-person Hands-on Healing of any kind
        before? When? Where? Results:

(40).   Have you ever tried Long-Distance Healing before? When? Where?
        Results:

(41).   Why did you choose to try DH? How did you choose a healer?

(42).   Did you believe that DH works before your healing? Why?

(43).   Has anyone you know received benefits from a DH treatment?
        Did this encourage you to try it?

(44).   To receive benefits from a DH, what do you believe is necessary?
        Why? (check all that apply)
        I have to be a good person to earn it from God
        I have to be going to church regularly
        I have to be praying, meditating, etc.
        I have to want it by Free Will
        Healing is a gift from God, all I have to do is receive willingly
        I have to act in accord with my desire to embrace health and
        Wholeness
        I have to see myself as being well, that healing can really happen
        I don't have to believe anything, it will be all done for me
        Faith
        I don't know
        Other:

(45)   If you do not receive benefits from a DH, what do you believe the
        barrier is? (check all that apply)
        God wants me to suffer because I need to be chastised
        illness is a lesson, I haven't learned what I need to know yet
        "karma" from a previous life.
        I am suffering instead of my children, family; I am taking on
        illnesses for their protection.
        I don't really want to be healed, life is too hard, I would rather be

156

sick or die.

I would lose all the attention my family and friends give me if I were well and healthy.

the time isn't right, healing will come at a later date

the devil or demons want me to be sick

I have a curse, spell, hex, generational bondage placed on me

I don't know

Other:

(46) In your opinion, why do people get sick? (check all that apply)

emotional stress causes physical problems

genetics inherited from relatives

poor eating habits and lack of exercise

no reason, the body just breaks down over time

chemicals in our food and water

military "chem-trails," government conspiracy, etc.

Other:

(47). In your opinion, how do you think DH works?

a universal source is doing the healing

a personal God is doing the healing

my higher self is doing the healing

the healer is doing the healing

hypnosis or mind control

mind over matter, client's power of positive thinking

I don't know

Other:

(48). Was the healing scheduled by you or by someone else, in your behalf? Why?

DURING THE DISTANT HEALING

(49). At the time of placing a request to schedule a healing, did you experience:

Noticeable difference in physical/emotional wellness after speaking with the healer

Noticeable difference in wellness after hearing the healer's phone message

157

No difference at all
I do not remember
Other:

(50). Your normal sleeping patterns: (check all that apply)
I sleep alone in my bed
I sleep with someone
There are other people in my house (children, etc)
There are pets in my house
There is no other living being in my house
I sleep very well
I sleep moderately well
I have difficulty in getting to sleep
I have difficulty staying asleep
Other:

(51). Were your sleep patterns any different on the night of the healing? If so, how?

(52). Did you wake up during the DH? (if yes, check all that apply)
I was not aware of any unusual event or feeling, everything was as normal
I felt I was not alone
I felt a warm sensation in my body (list where)
I felt a tingling sensation in my body (list where)
Did you see any mist, apparitions, or images in the room?
Did you see an image of Christ, Angels, or any religious figure in the room? Who?
Did you see an image of the healer in the room? Who?
Did any of these images appear as solid?
Did you hear any unusual sounds during the DH? What?
Did you smell any unusual odors during the DH? (Sweet/ Sour) What?
Other:

(53). Did you dream the night of the healing? Do you normally remember your dreams? If so, please describe:

AFTER EFFECTS OF DISTANT HEALING

(54). Upon awakening the next day, did you notice anything immediately different about your physical, emotional or spiritual state? What?

(55). Within the next 72 hours, did you notice anything different? What?

(56). Has there been noticeable changes in your condition in the time period beyond this time? (be specific, days, weeks, months?)

(57). Do you believe your DH experience affected how quickly or how fully you recovered from an illness or injury? Why?

(58). Have you been back to any health professional after your DH? Has there been a medical validation of results? If so, what?

(59). Overall, do you feel the DH affected your <u>physical</u> health?
Yes! I am completely healed of all ailments
Yes, I am healed of many of my ailments
I am healed of one or more of my ailments
I am not healed of any ailments
I do not know at this time

(60). Overall, do you feel the DH affected your <u>mental</u> health?
Yes! I am completely healed of all ailments
Yes, I am healed of many of my ailments
I am healed of one or more of my ailments
I am not healed of any ailments
I do not know at this time

(61). Overall, has the DH affected your <u>spiritual</u> health in any way? How?

(62). Has your experience with DH changed your belief in healing in any way? Why?

(63). If you were given Medical Intuitive/<u>Physical health</u> notes by the healer after the DH treatment, were they accurate?
Yes! Completely accurate!
Most of the medical information was accurate
Two or more details of the medical information was accurate.
Only one detail of the medical information was accurate
None of the medical information was accurate
I do not know yet. I have yet to be checked by a medical professional.
I told the healer everything before hand. Nothing was new.
Other:

(64). If you were given Medical Intuitive/<u>Emotional health</u> notes by the healer after the DH treatment, were they accurate?

Yes! Completely accurate!

Most of the emotional information was accurate

Two or more details of the emotional information was accurate.

Only one detail of the emotional information was accurate

None of the emotional information was accurate

I do not know yet. I have yet to be checked by a mental health professional.

I told the healer everything before hand. Nothing was new.

Other:

(65).   If you were given Additional Intuitive notes by the healer after the DH treatment, did they include:

Words, image or contact from someone who had died? (relatives/friends, etc.

Could you   recognize these people, did it seem accurate?)

Words, image or contact from God?

Words, image or contact from someone still alive?

Words, image or contact from pets who had died?

Words, image or contact from Saints or religious figures

Visions of items, places, homes that were recognizable and known to you?

Other:(accuracy level?)

(66).   Overall, in your opinion what was the most beneficial results from the DH? Why?

Physical healing

Emotional/mental healing

Spiritual healing

Medical intuitive/physical health notes

Medical intuitive/emotional health notes

Additional intuitive notes

Unknown yet

There were no benefits

(67).   Would you recommend DH to others as a integrative medicine?

Yes! There are benefits from distant healing

I don't know yet.

No, I don't think it works.

(68).   On a scale of 1-10, *(1 being min.(bad) 10 being max.(good)*

Please describe your general state of health, before and after the DH:

Pain: Before_____
After_____

Amount/Frequency of Medication	Before_____	After_____
Physical Activity/Energy Level	Before_____	After_____
Sexual Desire/Ability:	Before_____	After_____
Mobility and Flexibility:	Before_____	After_____
Ability to Sleep Well:	Before_____	After_____
Level of Anxiety & Stress:	Before_____	After_____
Happiness and Joy:	Before_____	After_____
Peacefulness, Tranquility:	Before_____	After_____
Spiritual Awareness:	Before_____	After_____
Other:_____	Before_____	After_____

(69). Did your experience with DH change: (circle one)

Your desire to help others?	Increased / No change / Decreased
Your interest in psychic phenomena?	Increased / No change / Decreased
Your concern with spiritual matters?	Increased / No change / Decreased
Your understanding of yourself?	Increased / No change / Decreased
Belief in a power greater than yourself?	Increased / No change / Decreased
Your personal feelings of self-worth?	Increased / No change / Decreased
Your tendency to pray?	Increased / No change / Decreased
Interest in science & quantum physics?	Increased / No change / Decreased
Interest in various forms of healing?	Increased / No change / Decreased

(70). Please write a description of your DH and tell anything else you would like to share (use more sheets as needed):

END – This concludes the Distant Healing Questionnaire.
Thank you for your time and support of this project!

RESULTS FROM THE RESEARCH QUESTIONNIARE:

I will leave the reader to draw their own conclusions from the information obtained. This basic statistical study will help show you overall group results. Whereas having all the research in front of me helps to answer such questions such as: "What percentages of seriously ill people receive a significant physical healing in relation to emotional healing, and are these immediate or long-term?" Many of these conclusions are submitted throughout the text of this book, in a form that may not be easily found here. Some of the wording of the questions are shortened - for the full question asked of the client, refer to the original questionnaire above. "N/A" means "Not Available," no answer was listed.

(1, 2).   216 clients participated in the study.

(3,11).   Ages - Between 21-87 years of age.

(4).   Sex - (83%) Female

(5,6).   Global - Clients from all over the world participated.

(7).   Marital Status - Divorced (41%) Married (28%) Single (24%) Widowed (7%)

(8).   Race - Caucasian (69%) Hispanic (4%) Native American (0%) Asian (3%) African-American (12%) Other (12%)

(9,10). Highest Level of Education completed: College over 2yrs (62%) High School (28%) Other (10%) *(NOTE - PhDs & MAs are listed as "College over 2 years," "Other" includes those who dropped out of college, went to technical schools, or those few who did not have any formal education, etc. This question may be viewed simply by seeing that most people who sought DH were well educated. Their occupations reflected this)*

(12).   Month & Year of DH:
         Conducted between spring 2004 - summer 2005.

(13).   State & Country DH occurred in: Global - Most people still lived in general proximity (within 200 hundred miles) to where they were born.(73%)

162

(14).   Condition of PHYSICAL health prior to DH: Moderate Health
         (50%) Seriously ill (32%) Experienced serious problem within 1 yr
         previously of DH (12%) Excellent health (6%)

(15).   Physical Condition diagnosed by a doctor: YES (79%) NO (21%)

(16, 17 18). Physical problems, length of time ill, family history: *These
         questions help with many of the conclusions referenced throughout
         the book. Listed in a group format would not be of benefit here. In
         most cases family history was -unknown.*

(19).   Substances taken within 48 hrs prior to DH: *(listed by category,
         clients were asked to mark all that applied. This question has a "no
         entry" percentage of (18%)* Stimulants (65%) Non-prescription (52%)
         Prescription drugs (48%) Alcohol (33%) Pain-killers (31%) Sedatives
         (22%) Hallucinogenic (4%)

(20).   Smoke? NO (81%) YES (19%)

(21).   Exercise? How often and what kind? YES (85%) NO (15%)
         *This figure is high because most people are trying to walk or stretch
         moderately often. Very few have a consistent or rigorous exercise
         program, health reasons often cited.*

(22).   Condition of MENTAL health prior to DH: Moderate Health
         (42%) Excellent Health (30%) Experienced serious problem within 1
         yr. previously of DH (18%) Seriously ill (10%)

(23).   Mental Condition diagnosed by a doctor: NO (87%) YES (13%)

(24, 25, 26). Emotional difficulties at time of DH, length of time ill, family
         history. *These questions help with many of the conclusions referenced
         throughout the book. Listed in a group format would not be of benefit
         here. Also, much of the family history was unknown.*

(27). Condition of SPIRITUAL health prior to DH: Excellent Health (45%) Moderate Health (38%) Other (17%) No interest in spiritual health (0%)

(28). What religion/spiritual path were you RAISED with? Protestant (35%) Catholic (29%) Other (19%) Eastern (8%) Jewish (6%) Agnostic (2%) Atheist (1%) Islamic (0%)

(29). What religion/spiritual path are you on NOW? *This was left open for the client to write in - when comparing this question with (28), most had left the path of their childhood (71%) yet many were still moderately involved with an "organized" faith (52%). With this question, a very large variety of spiritual paths were listed. Some examples were: esoteric, self-realized, Bhakta; many simply wrote in "spiritual" or "non-denominational Christian." N/A, blank entry or "still searching" (18%)*

(30). PRIOR to DH, how often did you attend religious/spiritual services? Holidays only (32%) Once a week (30%) Once a month (12%) Never (12%) Occasionally or Irregularly (8%) More than once a week (6%)

(31). AFTER your DH, how often did you attend religious/spiritual services? Once a week (32%) Holidays only (29%) Once a month (13%) Never (10%) Occasionally or Irregularly (8%) More than once a week (8%)

(32). Prior to your DH, did you routinely spend time doing any of the following? *(listed by category, clients were asked to mark all that applied. A "no entry" percentage of 22%)* Meditation (88%) Prayer (83%) Reading (80%) Exercise (79%) Nature (72%) Other (23%)

(33). After your DH, have any of these habits changed? NO (83%) YES (17%) *The percentage that changed unanimously a step in a beneficial direction. There were no changes toward bad habits listed.*

164

(34). Did you previously tell the healer what needed healing? YES (72%) NO (28%) Please list in detail what the complaints were: *This area was left open for the client to write in - each questionnaire was individually compared with #59, #60 and #63 #64. Most of the time (70%) what was listed here was vague - "physical healing," "emotional healing," etc. The remainder (30%) listed more specific needs.*

(35). Were you under any unusual stress, or undergoing life changes at time of DH? NO (82%) YES (18%)

(36). Tried CONVENTIONAL medicine or surgery before? YES (90%) NO (10%) Did it help? NO (77%) YES (23%)

(37). Special diet, supplements, nutrition plan? YES (68%) NO (32%)

(38). Tried ALTERNATIVE medicine or therapies before? YES (68%) NO (32%) Did it help? (81%) NO (19%)

(39). Tried IN-PERSON Hands-on Healing before? NO (73%) YES (27%) Did it help? YES (78%) NO (22%)

(40). Tried DISTANT HEALING before? YES (48%) NO (52%) Did previous healings help? YES (67%) NO (33%)

(41). WHY did you choose to try DH? HOW did you choose a healer? *This was left open for the client to write in. Most chose to try DH because they were curious or had a friend tell them about it. A variety of reasons were given on why they happened to chose me - the most common where these: a recommendation, reading one of my books, seeing me at a speaking event/healing convention, or internet search. Some other reasons cited for choosing me were: seeing me on a TV show or radio interview, Godly direction, personal intuition, because I was a Near-Death experiencer, etc.*

(42).	Did you believe DH works BEFORE your healing? YES (83%) NO (17%)

(43).	Has anyone you known received benefits from a DH? YES (51%) NO (49%)

(44).	To receive benefits from DH, what do you believe is necessary? *(listed by category, clients were asked to mark all that applied. This question has a "no entry" percentage of (2%).* Healing is a gift from God (90%) I have to want it by Free Will (72%) I have to act in accord with my desire to embrace health and wholeness (68%) Faith (25%) I have to see myself well (25%) I don't have to do anything, it will all be done for me (22%) I have to be praying, meditating, etc. (18%) Other (12%) I don't know (10%) I have to be going to church regularly (8%) I have to be a good person to earn it from God (5%)

(45).	If you do not receive benefits, what do you believe the barrier is? *(listed by category, clients were asked to mark all that applied. This question has a "no entry" percentage of (23%).* Time isn't right (38%)Don't know (33%) Lesson to be learned first (30%) Other (24%) Don't really want it (18%) Karma (17%) Curse (15%) Demons (14%) Loose attention from family (12%) Taking illness on myself instead of family (7%) I need to be chastised (3%)

(46).	In your opinion, why do people get sick? *(listed by category, clients were asked to mark all that applied. This question has a "no entry" percentage of (3%).* Emotional stress causes physical problems (92%) poor habits (86%) genetics (83%) chemicals (77%) body breaks down (68%) Other (21%) "Chem-trails" (7%)

(47).	In your opinion, how do you think DH works? *(listed by category, clients were asked to mark all that applied. This question has a "no entry" percentage of (1%).* Universal Source (89%) God (79%) Higher self (52%) Healer (42%) Mind over matter (33%) Other (30%) I don't know (29%) Hypnosis/mind control (11%)

(48).   Healing scheduled by you or someone else? Client (85%) Other (15%)

(49).   At the time of placing a request to <u>schedule</u> a healing, did you experience: No difference at all (55%) Noticeable difference in physical/emotional wellness after speaking with the healer (32%) Noticeable difference in wellness after hearing the healer's phone message (11%) I do not remember (2%) Other (0%)

(50).   Your normal sleeping patterns: *(listed by category, clients were asked to mark all that applied.* I sleep with someone (52%) I sleep alone (48%) I have pets in the house (48%) I sleep moderately well (43%) There are other people in my house - children, etc) (37%) I have difficulty in getting to sleep (34%) I have difficulty staying asleep (31%) Other (19%) There is no other living being in my house (17%) I sleep very well (12%)

(51).   Sleep patterns different on night of DH? NO (50%) YES (50%)

(52).   Did you wake up during the DH? YES (52%) NO (40%) If so, please continue: *(listed by category, clients were asked to mark all that applied. This question has a "no entry" percentage of (8%).* I felt a tingling sensation (72%) I felt a warm sensation (70%) I felt I was not alone (63%) I was not aware of any unusual feeling when I woke up (21%) Saw an image of the healer in the room (18%) Saw a mist, apparition, or image in the room (17%) saw an image of Christ, Angels, or other religious figure in the room (8%) Did any of these images appear as solid (NO 88%) YES (12%) hear any unusual sounds (12%) smell any unusual odors (10%) Other: (14%) *NOTE: "Other" included light in the room; disembodied arms or hands or face working over the body; seeing colors; hot sensations; animals acting strangely and waking the client up; and details of "unusual sounds"(i.e. voice calling   name) etc.*

(53).   Did you dream the night of the healing? YES (37%) NO (34%) N/A or I do not remember (29%)

(54).   Upon awakening the NEXT DAY, did you notice anything immediately different about your physical, emotional or spiritual state: YES (80%) NO (17%) N/A (3%)

(55).   Within the next 72 HOURS, did you notice anything different? YES (86%) NO (14%)

(56).   Has there been more noticeable changes in your condition in the time period *beyond* this time? YES (79%) NO (21%)

(57).   Do you believe your DH experience affected how quickly or how fully you recovered from an illness or injury? YES (64%) NO (12%) N/A (24%)

(58).   Have you been back to any health professional after your DH? Has there been a medical validation of results? YES (53%) NO (47%)

(59).   Overall, do you feel the DH affected your PHYSICAL health? YES (78%) NO (22%) Many ailments healed (33%) One or more ailments healed (30%) All ailments healed (15%) I don't know yet (12%) Not healed of any ailments (10%)

(60).   Overall, do you feel the DH affected your MENTAL health? YES (82%) NO (18%) Many ailments healed (37%) One or more ailments healed (30%) I don't know yet (14%) All ailments healed (15%) Not healed of any ailments (4%)

(61).   Overall, has the DH affected your SPIRITUAL health in any way? YES (71%) NO (22%) Don't know (7%)

(62).   Has your experience with DH changed your belief in healing in any way? How? *(NOTE: This question should have been worded differently - since some clients are coming from a place of belief, and some aren't. Change could mean going either way. Because of this,*

168

the answers to this question cannot be placed here in a bulk statistic.)

(63).   If you were given Medical Intuitive/*PHYSICAL HEALTH* notes by
the healer after the DH treatment, were they accurate? YES (86%)
NO (14%) Completely accurate (65%) Most was accurate (9%) Two
or more was accurate (7%) I do not know yet. I have yet to be
checked by a medical professional (6%) Only one detail of the
medical information was accurate (5%) I told the healer everything
beforehand. Nothing was new (4%) None of the medical information
was accurate (3%) N/A (1%)

(64).   If you were given Medical Intuitive/*EMOTIONAL HEALTH* notes
by the healer after the DH treatment, were they accurate? YES
(89%) NO (11%) Completely accurate (63%) Most was accurate
(11%) Two or more was accurate (8%) Only one detail of the
emotional information was accurate (7%) I told the healer everything
before hand. Nothing was new (5%) None of the emotional
information was accurate (4%) I do not know yet. I have yet to be
checked by a mental health professional (2%) Other (0%)

(65).   If you were given ADDITIONAL INTUITIVE notes by the healer
after the DH treatment, did they include: *(listed by category, clients
were asked to mark all that applied. This question has a "no entry"
percentage of (12%).* Words, image or contact from: someone who
had died (35%) Visions of items, places, homes (33%) Saints or
religious figures (21%) from God (19%) pets who had died (12%)
someone still alive (5%) Other (2%)

(66).   Overall, in your opinion what was the most beneficial results from
the DH? *(listed by category, clients were asked to mark all that
applied. This question has a "no entry" percentage of (3%).*
Emotional/mental healing (90%) Medical intuitive emotional health
notes (85%) Physical healing (83%) Medical intuitive/physical health
notes (79%) Additional intuitive notes (73%) Spiritual healing (58%)
Unknown yet (8%) There were no benefits (2%)

(67).   Would you recommend DH to others as a integrative medicine?
Yes! There are benefits from distant healing (92%) I don't know yet
(5%) No, I don't think it works (3%) N/A (0%)

(68).   On a scale of 1-10, *(1 being min.(bad) 10 being max.(good)* Please
describe your general state of health, before and after the DH:
NOTE: *These questions help with many of the conclusions referenced
throughout the book. Listed in a group format would not be of benefit
here, since clients entered on different levels than others. Overall
benefits of the DH were noted in all areas.* Pain, Amount/Frequency
of Medication, Physical Activity/Energy Level, Sexual
Desire/Ability, Mobility and Flexibility, Ability to Sleep Well, Level
of Anxiety & Stress, Happiness and Joy, Peacefulness, Tranquility,
Spiritual Awareness

(69).   Did your experience with DH change: *(NOTE: The answers to this
question cannot be placed here in a bulk statistic, since some clients
already had a healthy motivation in these matters, so would write "no
change." No Change could also reflect an entry where no beneficial
effect was noted. This would be answered by each questionnaire in its
entirety, and helps with the conclusions referenced throughout the
book.*

Increased / No change / Decreased (Circle One)

Your desire to help others?
Your interest in psychic phenomena?
Your concern with spiritual matters?
Your understanding of yourself?
Your belief in a power greater than yourself?
Your personal feelings of self-worth?
Your tendency to pray?
Your interest in science and quantum physics?
Your interest in various forms of healing?

(70).   Please write a description of your DH and tell anything else you would like to share (use more sheets as needed): *These questions help with many of the conclusions referenced throughout the book.* END of Distant Healing Research Questionnaire

Breaking it All Down

Let's look at some questions that were referenced earlier, and look at the results.

(1). Does age, culture or country the client lives in make a difference with the client's ability to benefit from distant healing? No, it does not seem to matter what age, background or part of the world the client is from. The statistics were consistently the same across the board. But we must note that there were entire countries that are not represented in this study, such as China and the USSR.

(2). Does sex of the client matter? Yes. Most of the clients were female, but it does look like sex may make a difference on how much healing is received by the client, and how it is perceived. The percentage of men that replied based a successful healing mostly on physical results, not on emotional or spiritual ones; whereas women regarded emotional and spiritual healing on the same benefit level as physical healing. Most of the women in the study are divorced white Caucasians with over two years of college. The second highest group was African-American females, and females who are currently married, and females who graduated from High School.

(3). How sick were they? Half of the clients had moderate physical health prior to the DH, the next highest group was seriously ill. In most cases, their condition had already been diagnosed by a doctor.

(4). Does alcohol or prescription drugs, non-prescription drugs (such as cold or allergy medications), sedatives, alcohol or stimulants (such as coffee and tea) make a difference in bodily receptiveness? How about smoking? This question applied to substances taken within 48 hours prior to the DH. A high percentage of people use some kind of stimulant, which includes coffee or tea. Over half use a non-prescription drug; with prescription drugs, alcohol and

pain-killers next highest on the list. Most of the clients did not smoke. And since almost all clients would recommend DH to a friend, and most received physical, emotional or spiritual healing, the answer would have to be NO, these factors did not influence the results of DH.

(5). Were they mentally stable? Yes. Only a small percentage were diagnosed with a mental condition by a medical doctor, half considered themselves to have moderate mental health, and the next highest percentage considered themselves in excellent mental health. From the questionnaires, there did seem to be a consistent correlation between the client and family history of depression, etc., when it was known.

(6). Does the client's religion, spiritual path, or lack of one play a role in healing? Half considered their spiritual health prior to DH as excellent, the next highest as moderate. There were none who had no interest in spiritual health. Most were raised Protestant, and secondarily, Catholic. Most had left the path of their childhood, yet half were still moderately involved with an organized faith, and some were still searching. Of those who go to church, the highest numbers prior to DH went to church only on holidays, yet the next highest percentage went consistently once a week. After the DH, there was a shift with these two numbers, with the highest percentage going to church consistently once a week, and the next highest only on holidays. In comparing the individual healing results with the questionnaire, there was a noticeable correlation between the client having some kind of spiritual path and the results that they were expecting, and the results they received. From all the numbers combined and based on no single religious/spiritual path, the results showed that most clients felt DH was an incentive for increased spiritual activities through a variety of means.

Just as a side-note here - I have seen that people who are more spiritually inclined receive healing better, unless their religious views emphasize that they should suffer. If they are at a place of forgiveness for themselves and others, which often comes within spiritual awareness, they are more apt to receive and see themselves as deserving of healing, and accepting of that. For Christians, that awareness includes their acknowledgement of their sins being forgiven and nailed to the cross. If a person continues to feel that they are

172

undeserving to be healed, and feels guilty for some reason, consistently the healing results will be far less for that person.

(7). _Does a distant healing change the emotional or spiritual habits of a person?_ Yes and No – most clients said the good habits were reinforced. The habits listed the highest were meditation, prayer and reading, followed closely by exercise and time with nature. It also increased interest in psychic phenomena, the desire to help others, and self-understanding.

(8). _Had most people already tried conventional medicine. Did it help with this problem?_ Yes, almost all had tried conventional medicine prior to DH. No, most believed it did not help. An equal number, over half, of clients were on a special diet, supplement or nutritional regime, and had tried alternative medicine before. And most clients felt the alternative therapies had helped them.

(9). _Do people have to believe that DH works, for it to actually work?_ Yes, the statistics show that most clients believed that it would work, and also that most people were healed. A conclusion might be drawn here, but a specific study is suggested focusing on intention and manifestation in these cases. Most people had never tried an in-person, hands-on healing before. About half had previously tried DH, and half had known someone who had benefited from it. Most chose to try DH because they were curious or had a friend tell them about it, and most of them scheduled the healing themselves.

(10). _What is the average person's belief about what a healing is and why a healing does or doesn't occur?_ Most clients believe that DH works from a universal source, and that it is also a gift from God, and that they have to want it and act in accord with it by embracing health and wholeness. If healing didn't work, most believed the time just wasn't right for it, and the next highest group didn't know any reason why healing wouldn't occur. Almost all believed people get sick because of emotional stress causing physical problems; with poor habits, genetics and chemicals being next highest on the list.

(11). Did clients know when the healing was going on? Yes. Over half of the clients woke up during the DH, with most of those feeling a tingling sensation or warmth in their body. Most felt they were not alone. Some were not aware of any unusual sensation when they work up, and some saw a mist, or an apparition image in the room. A small group saw an image of Christ, Angels, or another religious figure in the room. Most of these images did not appear to be solid, although some did appear that way. Some clients heard unusual sounds and odors of all varieties, and there were no negative or fearful sounds or odors listed. Many of them looked at their clock and made known the time of healing corresponded to the time of their unusual experiences.

(12). What percentage of clients receive immediate healings compared to in-process healing? Upon awakening the next day, most noticed a change in their physical, emotional or spiritual state. And in the next 3 days most clients noticed more of a difference, and in the time period beyond that, more noticeable changes in their condition occurred. Over half believed the DH affected how quickly they healed from an illness or injury (it wasn't stated how many had an injury or illness at the time), and about half have been back to their health professionals after their DH, with a medical validation of results. From individual questionnaires it can be noted that immediate, spontaneous healings occur just as frequently in DH as in in-person hands-on healing. This means full miraculous and spontaneous healing often occurred at the time that the healing was arranged for.

(13). How many received healing? Most people felt the DH positively affected their physical health, and many clients had many ailments healed. The same percentages held true for emotional healing.

(14). How accurate is physical and emotional medical intuition for DH? (This cannot be used as a standard across the board - since it depends on the method, connection and the healer. This could only be accurate with my results, with my methods, and through only one healer, me. BUT, this shows what can be accomplished, and also perhaps what degree of information is possible through remote viewing for medical intuition.) Most people had already told the healer what needed healing, but, only a very small percentage

174

(4%) stated that nothing was new. In other words, most people had told the healer what was needed, but received back much more information beyond what was given.

Most clients felt the accuracy of the notes given for physical medical intuition was very accurate, and well over half the group felt they were completely accurate. These stats held true for the emotional medical intuition as well. In addition, many who received additional information in the form of messages from the other side, such as loved ones, guides, God, religious figures, felt these were accurate. In areas where the intuitive notes contained information of visions of personal items, places, homes, etc., most felt these were accurate.

(15). Overall, what are the most beneficial results from a DH? Almost all felt the emotional/mental healing was the most beneficial result, with the emotional intuitive notes rated the next highest. Close behind is the benefits that came with the physical healing, and the physical intuitive notes. The additional intuitive information was also rated very highly as a benefit. Again, almost all would recommend DH to others as an integrative medicine, as most noted overall benefits with lessening of pain, increased energy levels, mobility and physical abilities. This includes a heightened sexual desire and ability, and lessening of anxiety and stress. Most felt an increase in joy, spiritual awareness, peacefulness and happiness.

CHAPTER 11
Bilocation - Sometimes People Will See You
When the Impossible Manifests Itself... Over & Over Again

Bilocation (BL) is an ancient phenomenon that dates back through the centuries. It has been experienced unexpectedly by the average person, and practiced through willful intent by mystics, saints, monks, yogis, and mystical adepts. There are certain ancient Biblical passages that possibly lend themselves either to levitation or bilocation; and indeed the long list of people adept at bilocation include St. Anthony of Padua, St. Ambrose of Milan, St. Severus of Ravenna, and St. Padre Pio of Italy, Maria Esperanza of Venezuela, Therese Neumann, Natuzza Evolo, St. Clement, St. Ambrose, Father Zlatko Sudac of Krk, Sister Maria Coronel de Agreda, and Teresa Higginson. Christian ascetics are not the only ones who claim the ability; texts relating bilocation appear in Hindu, Buddhist and Tantric literature, which include Sathya Sai Baba, and Paramahansa Yogananda, and Dadaji, among many others.

A typical example of bilocation is reflected in the story of St. Alfonzo: In 1774, St. Alfonso de'Ligouri was seen at the bedside of the dying Pope Clement XIV, when in fact the saint was confined to his cell in a location that was a four-day journey away. Those in attendance at the Pope's deathbed talked to Liguori, who lead them in prayers for the dying. Thus, Liguori's body appears to have been seen in two locations at the same time by multiple and reliable witnesses.

The list of known bilocaters is only partial - how many more are there that kept such delightful secrets to themselves, knowing that sharing such information would bring accusations of madness, blasphemy, mockery, or even witchery? How many reports were suppressed by the church of bilocation outside its own flock? How many people are there today, who still decide to keep quiet for religious, cultural or social reasons? Bilocation is much more common than once thought, both then and now; and when recognized, has a profound effect on those doing it, and those witnessing it. It

177

is truly a phenomenon that not only stretches the analytical mind, but rockets it through the envelope of our perceptions; shattering many concepts of reality along the way. It is an extreme experience that begs for description - yet, as is common with NDEs, stigmata and many OOBEs, no expressions or words exist that do it real justice.

Perhaps you are one who has experienced bilocation or knowingly witnessed it. You are not alone! There are many like us, and we desire to open the gates of acceptance for others. We are living in a wonderful age of information gathering and information sharing; and bilocation can be another wonderful tool for breaking the restraints of isolation and fear. Bilocation can bring the reality of the Divine supernatural into a world which has forgotten its ability and faith in going beyond what the physical body can do. This gives the average person something more *real* to hang on to. It is a life-changing and life-enhancing experience.

Some Personal Samples

"Thank you Tiffany, for visiting me in the hospital ICU. I was surprised because I was told only family could come to see me. Your smile and healing filled me with happiness and warmth! I went home sooner than expected, and I know I won't have to worry about complications. I'm sorry we couldn't talk, as you could see I had all those tubes. I thought you were in La Mesa on Wednesdays? But thank you for finding the time in your busy life to see me, it really meant a lot..." - T.M.

"...out of no where came this lady. I could not see her face, but she was dressed in a green-bluish medical clothing. Although I could not see her face, at that very moment I knew who it was. It was you - Tiffany! You calmly walked toward me and hugged me. I had this overwhelming sensation of well-being as a whole...you placed your right hand on the back of my head and your left hand on my right shoulder blade. Where your hands/fingers were placed, you slightly pressed down. Not only you knew what you were doing, but you knew exactly where your hands had to be. Very shortly thereafter, - where your hands were at - I felt a light tingling and warmth. The feeling was coming more from the tip of your fingers than from your whole hands. Most

178

importantly, my whole self entered a stage of total Peace. This Peace was not surrounding me, this Peace was located inside of me. I live in Canada, I know you could not really be here in my room. "What a beautiful dream," I said to myself...or was it? Throughout my whole "dream/experience" not one word has been spoken from neither of us. This whole experience was so overwhelming, that I consciously "woke-up" when you left, but didn't move...and I could still feel the warmth, tingling and light pressure of where your hands were! It has been the best experience/place I have ever been on this earth. Thank you Tiffany for visiting me! Just when I thought The Big Guy was done with me...Maybe there is hope for me after all! My home is always open to you..." - M.B.

"I saw you, and your voice is what woke me up! You were calling my name, and saying "the left side of your body, the left side, open up for healing on the left side..." I didn't feel afraid at all! The room was glowing blue, I could see your features very well, at first I thought you were an apparition, but now I don't think so, because you kept talking to me. How you do it, I don't know! It really freaked me out at first! But the real miracle is I HAVE NO PAIN this morning. I really know I've been healed! Do you know how big this is? No pain! I've been so mad at God, but today I felt peaceful. Clarence (my dog) saw you too, and started barking, I don't know if you saw him or not. I know God sent you. Now I'm going to look for you every time he barks..." - C.S.

"I just wanted to tell you, my mom is well this morning...we knew you did the healing last night, because mother woke up and saw a lady fitting your description (she's never even seen a picture of you!) wearing a long pink dress standing near her bed and singing. She wasn't afraid at all! You told her to "have faith...don't be fearful," then you touched her head and placed her hands at her side. The illness that has plagued my mother for over a year is now gone..." – V. M (NOTE: I was wearing a pink nightgown at the time of the BL)

What is Bilocation?

In the Merriam-Webster Dictionary, it is defined as:
Main Entry: bi·lo·ca·tion

Pronunciation: 'bI-lO-"kA-sh&n
Function: noun
Date: 1858:
the state of being or ability to be in two places at the same time
(Latin: *bis*, twice; *locatio*, place)
(or sometimes *tri* or *multi*location)

"Bilocation is the Illuminated Path of the Supreme Consciousness. It is the secret way that all masters use to reach the ultimate of all universes. One must learn the separation of spirit from body by his own volition. It increases awareness, helps solve problems and gives a spiritual insight into one's own Akashic records and the hidden worlds." - Paul Twitchell, *Orion Magazine*

"When an adept bilocates, they will participate at a personal and individual level. When in this state, it is possible to maintain concurrent conscious awareness in both bodies simultaneously. One is, in fact, in two places at the same moment with their full awareness intact, a "splitting" or "multiplication" of awareness." - Rawn Clark, *A Bardon Companion*

Sounds like an OOBE, doesn't it? Or maybe even RV - but BL is neither of these two things, even though people often interchange the words haphazardly. *But bilocation is a different mechanism.* It takes *both* of these things to allow yourself to come to a place of total immersion. *The mechanics of what we are as energetic Divine creatures is nowhere more evident than when doing this sort of work.*

I will give you research information and personal experience in this chapter about bilocation, but you alone will be left to discern the subtle nuances of these levels of consciousness. I feel the true freedom of understanding will be the desire and practice of *experiencing* these gifts on your own merits. In this way, conscious knowing will make up the gap where the written word has once again failed. In my thoughts, the word "bilocation" is a limiting misnomer anyway - since a multitude of simultaneous locations can be accessed at once, into several different parts, all a reflection of the original - a true holographic representation of unity in each piece of the one.

180

"The thing that distinguishes this from normal imagination is the uninterrupted or continuous nature of the inner experience and its clarity or three-dimensional quality. In this kind of spiritual travel, the experiencer can instantaneously shift back to the physical senses with no resistance or time required to regain normal waking sensory experience. This kind of spiritual travel is perhaps a more advanced form since it allows for integration of inner and outer experience...The shift between the two can take place anywhere...This shift back and forth between two completely separate existences, one in the body and one out of the body is...the ability to perceive two separate worlds." - J. Denosky, *Spiritual Travel*

"BILOCATION - This is where the Consciousness, the Astral body, the Etheric body & the Physical body are in TWO different places at the same time. This is only to be used by advanced Magi and then rarely. It involves time & place distortion with a host of other things." - Angelfire.com *Astral Projection*

Bilocation Already a Reality in Quantum Physics - the "Padre" Electron

What some consider rare in our macroscopic reality, is a factual everyday occurrence in the atomic and sub-atomic world of quantum physics. Whether you were first exposed to bilocating electrons through movies such as *"What the Bleep Do We Know?"* or through higher mathematics at University, what we couldn't believe could possibly exist was there all along! And science, as we have seen throughout this book, is learning more all the time.

"Atoms and sub-atomic particles can be in many places at ones. And we can prove it! During the early half of the 20th century, scientists came to realize that electrons themselves, as well as other atomic and sub-atomic particles may be considered as both particles and waves. In fact if you shoot electrons through two slits (as we did with light) then a similar interference pattern of dark and light fringes will be produced. The surprise came when scientists realized that the same interference pattern will be produced even if a single electron is shot through the two slits! Now, electrons must be passing from both slits at the same time, if they are to interfere with each other and produce an interference pattern. So a single electron must be at both slits

181

(i.e. at different places) at the same time! That's what we call bilocation and what we usually associate with mystics and the supernatural. And it is the most natural experience for the electron, for the packets of light, as well as for other atomic and subatomic particles!" - The "Padre" Electron and The Breathtaking Quantum View(s) Of The Universe by Prof. Victor Axiak

Bilocation is Not Remote Viewing

"I have been doing CRV (controlled remote viewing) for over 14 years...in all those years, the "bilocation" experience has only happened to me about 9 or 10 times...in CRV, the "bilocation" state is actually discouraged because when you begin experiencing the target fully, you are no longer aware of the monitor and pen and paper in front of you. When you finish the experience, all you can do is give the best summary you can come up with. Then, you are dependant on your memory, your biases, etc. - a process which is extremely prone to error and gross misinterpretation...the CRVer works progressively from vague, random thoughts, through daydream-type impressions, through very realistic impressions, and can possibly work up to the point where it APPEARS to the viewer that he/she is actually at the target site (CRV is NEVER the same as an out of body experience)." Lyn Buchanan - Controlled Remote Viewing Canada

Similar to a RV, bilocation can be accomplished while mentally awake, yet in a meditative and deeply quiet mode, and focused at the "out-bound" site. As noted above, bilocation is not good for the tasks of RV, since you are "experiencing the target fully" and not able to utilize any note taking instruments or to vocalize what you are seeing.

If RV is a 50/50 split consciousness, and OOBE is 98/2 (the silver-strand still intact), I would guess that BL (a term I'll coin here for "bilocation") is more like 150% consciousness *there*, while 50% consciousness is razor-sharp *here* to help control the intent. It doesn't make sense to the logical mind, does it! I find that mostly the physical "home" body is left in free-form mode (which may be paralyzed for some people but "on automatic" with others) which is only partially ignored by the out-bound body.

182

Bilocation is Not Lucid Dreaming

If you experience any of the lucid dreaming states, such as the ability to change things in your surreal surroundings as you desire, *you are not bilocating*. If you look at your hands or feet and they fade away or look elongated, *you are not bilocating*. Bilocation is not a dream. It is real, and you will be able to readily find these facts as you experience it. *"In nine of Natuzza Evolo's bilocations, she left bloodstains at the scene...Padre Pio left a hand print on glass that could never be wiped off, and five times bloodstains from his stigmata...Maria de Agreda, a cloistered Franciscan nun who evAngelized natives through bilocation in Spain and Mexico, distributed rosaries there which disappeared from her home cell."* - The PK *Zone* by Pamela Rae Heath MD

If you can eat (though it tastes like cardboard), run into doors instead of going through them and clearly see numbers, read clocks, and have forward-focused vision only, then you are bilocating. If you feel heavy and experience the effects of gravity, you are bilocating. And yes, people can interact with you, and you with them; and you can feel pain. I have come back with bruises before, and cuts and scrapes that manifested on my outward home body; I do not know how or why this happens. One must be careful when bilocating, and treat the out-bound body gently.

Bilocation is Not an Out-of-Body Experience

In every OOBE that I have had, I have only been vaguely aware of the physical body I left behind. If you have *not* read the previous chapters on Out of Body or Remote Viewing, I suggest you review them now; I want you to clearly see the differences, and that's why this chapter comes later in the book. With the OOBE, I take myself down to the lowest possible heart rate, slowing my breathing to the point of sleep in my body, and indeed my arms and legs, etc. come into a paralyzed state. My point of consciousness goes out, either from the top of my head or belly. I separate completely into the projectable double. With an intentional BL, at some point the double becomes entangled with the physical, yet not in proximity to it - an adrenaline rush is felt, and full awareness, sometimes pain, and a dizzying effect of "puppeting" from one

183

time in another, and weightiness. At first the light is blinding, and it takes a bit to get your balance and bearings; it is almost like zooming through the NDE tunnel of bright light.

In an OOBE, only if my physical body signals *something is wrong* will I be reminded to return to the body before I would have chosen to. Yet with BL, I am still aware of my physical body, as in RV, and I am conscious of arms, legs, etc. But, I am also totally absorbed in the other dimension, and indeed, feel like my body walking *there* is walking *here,* as if the nervous system is firing commands to this body that makes my "other" body move. It is as if the energy here is needed to stimulate activity there; I cannot fully escape the body when doing a bilocation, it feels in some way I need it as a 'stand in' for my other half. Perhaps the need is just a human thing for grounding, or a touch-stone for real-time, I really don't know. Also, I have *never* noted any bilocation to occur beyond *real-time* mode; this is not the case with RV and OOBE, which can indent through time and dimensions effortlessly.

Perhaps a good example is a TV screen with "picture within a picture" mode, a mini-picture of one channel up in the corner going on as normal, while the "other" is fully occupying the larger screen. Yet, both are operated by one control unit, which in this case would be the consciousness of the one doing the bilocation, and in all BL cases that I know of, the Greater Consciousness as well. How to put BL in a nut-shell? OK, here goes: *"Bilocation is real-time controlled remote viewing, in a fully unconscious out of body experience, powered by self intent and Divine uumph!"*

Do Only Holy People Bilocate?

If one definition of "holy" means that every motivation for the event comes from a deep sacred place of abiding love or passion, then from everything that I can see, the simple answer would be *"Yes."* Why would this be the case? *Because the energy required to bilocate is beyond what the astral or etheric bodies can produce on their own.* An Energy Source beyond one's own capability is required, *a Sacred Power Connection.* It also seems the person who is able to still one's mind to the point of willful (not spontaneous) bilocation must of necessity long ago released any lower vibrations of negative

184

emotions or ego. Letting all other things go, he has chosen to advance himself to the highest frequency of clear-mindedness, peace, tranquility, and love. It in no way requires saint-hood, just a focused everyday intent of love for one another, Source, and ourselves; this in itself is sacred, or Holy.

In every case concerning myself, complete trust and surrender is absolutely necessary to relinquish oneself for benefit and concern of another. I have been able to "click out" with an OOBE or RV as I wish, to "look in" on friends and clients almost whenever I choose to by Free Will (unless I find a block on their side or from The Big Guy). But I have never been able to bilocate *without added help* and a *good purpose* to do so. For me, God is always in the picture with bilocation; and if He withholds His power from it, *it ain't gonna happen!* This has also been an excellent safeguard for me, and I have come to fully rely on it - in this way, I know that it isn't just "my idea," and the event has merit for its occurrence. Therefore, I don't need to worry about anything, and can give it my all; because I know it is all for the highest possible good - or else it wouldn't occur.

This also lets me relax into Love's call to bilocate to an unknown place that has been chosen. Sometimes this spontaneous calling also happens for an OOBE. But if *I am the one who chooses* to BL, I need an indent of some sort to find my way to, just like in RV and DH. For me, seeing a crisis on TV or in the newspaper can often stimulate enough of an emotional imprint for either RV, OOBE or BL. I have often remarked to myself that I am glad that I don't need much sleep at night, since I wouldn't have time for any more than that! There is so much to be done, places to go, people to help, and things to see; and all without waiting in airport terminal lines! Indeed, a good 100% of the bilocations I have experienced are when God chooses spontaneously where and when, and my only need is to open my intention to fully comply, and away we fly.

"I only know that it is God Who sends me," replied Padre Pio when *questioned about it. "I do not know whether I am there with my soul or body, or both of them."* - Padre Pio: The True Story by C. Bernard Ruffin

The Energy Required to Bilocate

185

We can't see the bilocating electrons of our quantum world; the naked eye can't even see just the very small things in our universe, such as viruses and bacteria. But, modern man knows they are there, and science has proven many things that were considered "madness" in ancient times. For example, for hundreds of years man thought that blood ebbed and flowed in the veins like the tides of the sea; and of course, that the world was flat! We have come such a long way from those days of ignorance. Or have we?

If we are truly honest about it, we really see that we are still in our infancy. In the new dimensions of M-strings and quantum mechanics, we are having to learn the reasons behind what is being already experienced; in many ways, we are working backwards from the end result to the mechanics of "why?" This can be a daunting task. But, with so many students eagerly flocking to the new physics, many profound discoveries are sure to be found in the next few years. And I dare say the relationship between science and spirituality will grow fonder and more compatible as truth is revealed.

But, does knowing "how" something works increase our ability to operate it better? Perhaps. Similar to knowing how a car mechanically operates; the driver has all the technical knowledge available on what makes it travel down the road, and the driver may be able to make more informed guesses about unfamiliar noises when they occur. But that doesn't change the fact that you still have to do all the things the "uninformed" person has to do - pump the gas, check the oil, air filter, brakes, tires, etc. Regular maintenance is necessary to keep the car running smoothly as a consistent tool to get from here to there. So it is with exploring, and accessing all of these dimensions we are talking about. We don't have to be "universe mechanics" or scholars to experience these lovely avenues of advancement for ourselves, and to contribute to the enrichment of others, but there does seem to be the basics to learn.

One more question - what happens if the user of the car doesn't fill the gas tank? Something as simple as that stops the entire equation from working, and it doesn't matter if you technically know what causes compression in the engine or not. It is the same with BL, and indeed with OOB and RV too.

186

Without power, nothing will occur. Now, this is the important part - bilocation takes a terrific amount of power - a space rocket cannot be compared to a 757 passenger plane. Remote viewing and producing out-of-body experiences can be done on a person's own will and power (though I don't suggest it), on one's own gasoline - it is: *"My will be done."* Bilocation is: *"Thy will be done."*

Trusting in the event being real, and that no true harm will befall you, is like premium gasoline in the tank, with fuel injection and 32 pistons cranking under the hood. As in a healing event when we see the person whole and well in our mind's eye and bring them to that place of spiritual entrainment where anything and everything can happen, so in BL we begin with the same kind of faith. And *faith* is what it is, according to the Biblical definition:

"Now faith is being sure of what we hope for, being certain of what we cannot see." (Heb. 11:1, NIV) or *"Faith is the assured expectation of what is hoped for though not beheld."* (NW)

Similar to the ancient Israelites who were given numerous laws by Moses that they had no logical reason to believe, such as: burying their excrement outside the camp; washing up to their elbows after touching dead bodies and other 'unclean' things; burning the clothes and personal items of leprous and diseased people; etc. These ancient people knew nothing of germs. They just had faith. And when they worked in accord with it, they prospered while the other nations around them died off of 'unknown' plagues and diseases. We may not know all the 'hows' and 'whys' of bilocation, but it really doesn't need to be an analytical thing. Much of it will always remain a mystery anyway, since the Power to do it is always teaching yet can never fully be known. It is a heart thing, and seeing it real creates faith, and a successful and fulfilling experience.

When bilocation first started happening, I nervously told a colleague and friend of mine, who happens to be an unconventional and enlightened Catholic priest. His reply? A warm smile and truthful words of advice: *"Stop analyzing it and just enjoy!"*

Sometimes You Won't Realize You are Being Seen – My First BL

"Sometimes I know where I go, but other times I don't. I find out because someone sees me and tells me." - Maria Esperanza , *The Bridge to Heaven* by Michael H. Brown

So how does it happen that sometimes you will be RV or OOB and all of a sudden a bilocation happens? Because your intent and desire is so strong, and you cross into an entangled state of consciousness, *and then The Big Guy plugs you in.* Whatever you were working on just got a higher priority, and you're now being fully utilized to be in the right place at the right time, and everything changes! This was how I was awakened to the reality of bilocation. Everyone will have a different story, but with me, there was also a bit of a preamble before the big event!

Normally, before a distant healing, I feel very clear on my remote viewing aspects, and sometimes I note to my secretary the details of the room and the house the client lives in, as well as the layout of the neighborhood, the weather, etc. During this time the medical intuition is done (during 50/50 RV split time). Then I consciously "let go" of the body and go into the out-of-body healing mode, which means I wouldn't be able to talk anymore, but would be able to be a clearer channel for Holy Spirit to work for healing (98/2 OOB). From there, I would be able to let the client's body "glow" and saturate all the high vibratory goodness for wholeness and balance. Then, when The Big Guy was done, I could either "go play" in real-time around the location area and explore; go elsewhere in dimension and explore; or come back home, go into sleep and wake up the next morning. But this next time would be different; my first bilocation.

During my Sabbatical times, I do not do any distant healings, although I will schedule them for when I come off the Sabbatical. One night, I was at my desk writing, my body went through the physical steps of OOB; being paralyzed, etc, but with no sense of "coming or going." Then from the paralyzed feeling I immediately found myself standing at the bedside of a client who was about 1,500 miles away, though I didn't know it at the time. This person was scheduled for a distant healing the next month; this was going

188

to be a spontaneous bilocation healing. When I found myself at the bedside, I had no idea where I was, or who he was! But, I thought I might as well heal while I was here, since that is usually the purpose for me to be anywhere. I would try to figure it all out later, and why I felt so different this time.

It was at this moment, when I decided to start the healing, that the person woke up with a start and turned and looked straight at me. He quickly sat up in bed, met me eye to eye, and screamed! *He saw me!* It shocked me *out of my skin!* And fear, of course, this makes you jump back into your body (I guess it shocked me *into* my skin?) - and I exploded back so fast that I came back "wrong" and I spent over an hour not being able to focus right and stumbling around and physically walking into walls! What had just happened?! Was this just a dream, why did things feel so different, and how was it that a person could look me in the eye? It was so confusing! Also, why was I so out of sync that I had to "click out" again with an OOBE, and come back correctly? This took some time to do, since my heart and mind was racing about what had just happened.

Up to this time, numerous people had mentioned unusual things during distant healings - seeing apparitions or ghostly images of loved ones, other people, of me or even religious saints. All this had made me wonder about the conscious and subconscious perceptions of the clients. Was it a psychic event that required their own ability to be sensitive? How much and what they were actually seeing? But, before this night, I had never had physical *interaction* eye to eye, or felt the strange way I did.

I was trying to figure all this out during the day, wondering what the reaction of the man would be, who he was, and if what I had experienced was truly real. I had a pretty good hunch it was someone who had requested me for a healing, but beyond that, I had no idea. So, I decided to leave it alone. I nervously checked my messages several times during the day, thinking that if the person knew me or had any connection with me, that I would get an email. Then, I went to my computer, and there it was, an email there waiting for me; from the man I had "seen," or rather, had "seen" me.

"Dear Tiffany: Thank you for the healing! This morning I woke up without

189

any pain, and this after so many years of suffering and medication. I need to tell you I really didn't believe, and only tried it because of (my wife's) prodding. But then an Angel appeared to me last night, and now I know anything can happen. After it left, I felt so hot I had to kick off the covers, and I could feel things happening inside me. Then I slept the best sleep I've had in years. I'm not sure I understand all this. But I am thankful."

It was a man who had been scheduled for distant healing several weeks later. I wrote him back, asking for details about what the "Angel" looked like, and encouraged him to validate the healing with a medical follow-up as soon as possible. I just had to shake my head and wonder. A myriad of thoughts went through my head – was this some kind of weird 'parallel dreaming?' I needed to know more.

"Dear Tiffany: It was very close to my face, right by my bed…when I saw it, it disappeared, its eyes were very big. It looked like a real woman with pale skin, which seemed to glow…it had a flowing blue dress on…after it left the night was purple around my bed instead of black…"

My heart stopped in my chest - last night, I had been wearing a long blue nightgown! And definitely my eyes would have been big! I emailed him back and said:

"Signs and wonders never cease! God gave you the ability to see me (sorry, not an Angel!) and gave you the healing (not me, but Him!) to help get you to a place of awareness of the reality of the impossible, and bring you to a place of openness where you can accept the supernatural Love and Care He has for you. You surprised me when you saw me – I heard you scream! Did you hear me? That was my blue nightgown I had on. You are right, everything is possible; but only when we open ourselves to that opportunity, which has occurred here…I know you will continue to be Blessed and more open to Spirit and healing than ever before…there are real Angels too, I just want you to know…"

His reply…*"Dear Tiffany! Yes! I heard screaming and only part of it was me! I had wondered about that, since I didn't think Angels would do that...this has really opened a can of worms I closed a long time ago...I might have some questions..."*

Further follow-up has shown complete physical recovery in this case, and a great stimulation to venture upon the spiritual path, an awakening of answers with his "can of worms." It was my awakening too! Another kind of "lighting-strike," as the reality of this new awareness felt like I was going crazy - as the reasoning analytical brain said "this is not possible!" and turned inside out to grasp this experience.

In this case, it seemed enough of a physical manifestation for vocal cords to operate, and nuances of skin and fabric colors to be seen, although no physical manipulation of objects or touching occurred. I believe some manifestations may not come into complete material form - it may be hard to know in some cases how much matter is physically materialized at any given time. One of the best ways to know is to try to do "normal" things, and to receive validation from others who see you.

A Person Bilocating Can Do Many Normal Things

At least in the beginning, I would say this is the best way that you will be able to know that you are actually bilocating; is that someone sees you. With only a partial manifestation, there seems to be "onion layers" of subtleties with how it "feels" to your perceptions as you experience it. Until then, you will have to rely on outside validation to prove that you have manifested enough to be seen, and to break that through that ceiling of supposed reality in your head! A *full* manifestation comes naturally with the memory of all of your regular habits - how to hold things, walk, and even to eat and converse. A person bilocating can do many normal things and have a sensation that it is actually occurring, though it feels different in many ways.

When I have tested out bilocation with people who know me well and see me often, some have asked: *"How are you feeling today?"* The report has been to the effect that I seemed different, seemed distracted, dazed or *"out of it,"* or didn't converse at all or very little. Like I *wasn't all there (ha!)*. I don't

191

know if this will improve with time or not, or if it is just characteristic of the nature of bilocation, or perhaps just of my own limitations.

I have long witnessed that animals (especially cats) and small children will sense me when I am astrally out of body, and it seems they respond differently to me when I am bilocating too. Animals are very sensitive to changes in spirit in all forms.

I have found that in order to do BL *intentionally,* you must have an innate grasp of the nature of Free Will and have consistently worked with Divine energy before. You must completely trust and surrender that the highest good will happen with each event; keep yourself on a high frequency level of clean and clear mind and body; and last but not least, you must have control over your own intent and a keen desire to help others with unconditional love, then ask Father, and there you go...!

Folding Space & Time, Indenting a Connection
Five Logical Steps to Bilocation, What it Feels Like

What follows is only my experience; I do not pretend to know what every bilocater feels, this is just my own story. In my research, I actually couldn't find any first-hand descriptions of this modality - perhaps this is the first recorded one. But this description is simply offered as a student's weak pencil drawing of a delicate and detailed full-color Old Master oil painting. This is just my perception, but offered as empirical experience nonetheless, learned at the point of impact.

When a bilocation happens, the sudden rush of Energy makes me feel instantly nauseated, an adrenaline rush happens, and immediately I am *at* the location (unless I was already there, as in a distant healing). It is not like the somewhat slower *going* to the location like an OOBE. In my nausea, I immediately *sink* and feel like an atmosphere (30 ft.) of water is on top of me, and I'm at the bottom of a very deep pool. My eyes, hearing, and sense of smell feel slow and groggy, there is a bright light, and I have to focus very hard on bringing everything up to speed. My eyes are never as totally clear as my home body vision, though my hearing becomes quite sensitive. I start to feel my skin and the sparks of activity move what feels like chemical and nerve pulses down my body, and I move my head and look around. It could be that the impulses in my home body are what I am feeling, or it is being mimicked, I do not know.

Most of the time I have the sensation of a headache that pounds all the way through it - I have learned to view this as a safeguard to help me know the difference between worlds, and to keep one foot in my home body. As I mentioned before, BL seems to have a much higher need for physical connection than in an OOBE.

When I realize what has happened, and I am steady enough, I start asking all the questions in my mind, that I need to know. In a spontaneous BL, there will be plenty! "Who am I here for? Where am I? What should I do now?" and The

Big Guy will choose to answer them, or not. There is always a purpose, and I go about my business, and it will unfold as His Will, My Will, and Free Will allows. Often the answers will be general and simple, "the first door, knock there," "the child that comes up to you, him," "the Middle East," etc.

By this time I am totally absorbed into the new experience, and only vaguely aware of my home body, which is usually slumped into a chair, at the desk, or outside in the countryside. Sometimes my home body will go into a slow movement that repeats itself (one time I rubbed my right eyebrow off), but most of the time it seems still. My home body always seems exceptionally warm to me during this time, and my face always looks flushed when I return. I also have to lie down and sleep afterwards, no matter what time of day it is. Evidently it takes a lot of work on my body's to sustain what is occurring. Sometimes I will write down the information about the bilocation before I lie down to sleep, but if I don't, it is always there when I wake up - which is much clearer than an OOBE memory would ever be, and better than RV too. The sleep is very sound, and often for 8-10 hours! Since my normal sleeping pattern has been much less than that, this is a lot of recuperation for me!

When I wake up, there is more physical regeneration/recuperation that occurs over the next 24-48 hours. On a physical level, my skin will look very wrinkled and is very dry; it literally *takes something out of me physically* to do this. Sometimes there will be, for lack of a better term, some kind of "ectoplasm" that is left "gelled" on my skin. Also, after the long bilocations (which can be a few hours) or ones where there is a lot of interaction, often I will have blood clots in my nose. After every bilocation - the top of my head becomes very, very sensitive, where even brushing my hair or showering my head is painful. And, as I mentioned before, sometimes bruising or scrapes will be noticed on my physical body, and sometimes I will have diarrhea. As I brighten, these physical effects are lessening, and there seems to be less strain on my body and less recuperation time needed.

Also after BL, I crave salmon! Raw or medium-rare salmon, with lots of fresh dark greens, and a small handful of sunflower seeds. Nothing else will do! There must be something in these items my physical body needs. I make sure the fish is organic, hormone and chemical free, and only purchased from a natural foods store. With this kind of meal, and after the 24-48 hours, and rest, my skin will be soft and full again and all the wrinkles will be gone.

In readjusting to my home environment, I find the mind goes through a period of "frazzle," for no better term for it. I literally feel compelled to make sure I am in my home body - I spend time remembering the linear time-line of what I was doing yesterday, or the morning or evening leading up to the BL. I call friends and talk about casual things; I call the Institute and make sure the appointment schedule matches the one in my book. I play with the cats; I pull weeds in the garden; I do anything I can to feel "real" and grounded to this physical body and the earth around me. I need to feel "home" again.

Often, just for safety's sake, I won't drive until everything is more "normal." I probably have at least a portion in the back of my brain still wondering and making sure that I am really "here." Stupid questions initially floated through my mind about it; such as "what if this happens while I'm *driving!*" and "what if I *stay* wrinkled, and end up looking like an old woman the *rest of my life!*" But as I have learned in all my experiences with The Big Guy - just relax! He's the One in charge, and He hasn't taken all this time to train me up just to lose me now. There is purpose in all of it, and I am in it for the long run.

The Importance of Purpose

When I look at things during a bilocation, there is a bit of *overlay* on it in many ways that is different from *real* perception. It feels almost like I am drunk, if I move my head too quickly, things blur and I lose balance. I also feel lighter in comparison to my home body, and this makes me clumsy. I feel varying stages of pressure with gravity on this kind of body - and I gauge this as a key to "how much" I am manifesting. I think that I can safely measure the amount of pressure I feel with the gravitational pull of mass to the amount of physical manifestation. I try not to do anything stupid when in this state, since I don't want to accidentally train my home body to accept lack of controls in its real life. Unlike an OOBE, you are not going to jump off a cliff and try to fly, it would not be wise. Since I have injured it before, I really don't know how far this can go. If you "die" in a bilocation, does it transition to your home body? No. But, it is good to be careful just the same.

195

I learned early on with the OOBE that I needed to be very aware of what my home reality is and what it is not, or else I could lose my body before I am done with it, through shear stupidity in the "real" world! For example, in my home body and in real time, too many times I've been driving down a steep canyon road, or looking out from an ancient Anasazi cliff face and felt in my mind's eye the memory of my astral body stepping out into the beyond. If I didn't have a hold on what is here, and what is not, I could make some grave mistakes, literally. I need to make a sure and definite distinction between my home body and the other states. I suggest you do too. It is like knowing when you are dreaming, and when you are not. You must have safeguards in place or learn to never take chances – even in your dreams! What fun would that be? Not much!

It is important to find grounding within your home reality, and have borders in place just in case you forget what body you are in. I believe this is one reason why so many of the people we have stories from are also those who have a very high purpose, or mission, to accomplish yet in their life, so the desire to finish the job keeps them grounded enough to keep them coming back to their home body. I would say that because of all these dangers, that only the adept consciousness with advanced awareness transverse these dimensions - although it probably won't initially be up to you when you are brought into this experience anyway, at least the first time. But, you can prepare, and have better understanding now.

Balance Between the Worlds

In bilocation, I have been gone for as little as half an hour, and up to four hours at a time. As my experience was when I first started healing, I find it has taken time to build up to the sustained flow of increased outbound time with the body. Working with critical clients and desperate cases produces a rush too. I find my physical body can only take so much, and Father often encourages my progress by taking me right to the edge of the envelope. Right when I just can't see how I can possibly keep my finger in the 220 electrical socket anymore without exploding all the bulbs - and the building they're in too! Yet, taking me to the edge of my capability always magnifies where I

196

need to surrender more fully, and trust allows full compliance in Love.

When I am *stretched*, my head may feel like it is ready to burst, my eyes to pop out of their sockets, and there can be blood in my nose, and a sustained period of dizziness, stomach cramping, heart palpitations, and some stomach problems with this too. But, this stretching has consistently occurred periodically throughout my years of being facilitated for the normal healing work, and is short-term until my body adjusts and brightens to a new level. I am thankful for it, because the after-effects are long lasting and strong, allowing me to be a better Light connection from then on, and it helps me attain a new level of getting my own self out of the way. I become a larger and clearer conduit for more healing miracles.

Please note that you will not find many of my own excursions written here, since I feel these missions are under Divine direction and involves the privacy of others. The ones that are here are included just to show some feedback. The point is not to blow my own horn or make people wonder if the person they just had a healing with wasn't exactly "all there." I don't worry about it; it's a God thing.

This chapter is written to help you with *your* great mission, mine are mere examples. I am still learning in all things, just a simple little one in the woods following a golden butterfly. Everything here is about helping *you* ease into this opportunity for yourself, to know you are not alone, and perhaps to give you an idea of what to expect.

The Confusion of Words

"Apparitions of the Living: Also called bilocation, apparitions can be either spontaneous or intentional. In the case of spontaneous bilocation, the person whose apparition is seen is generally (though not always) unaware of his/her bilocation. Bilocation is considered intentional when the apparition can be connected to a person who was aware s/he was having an out of body experience (OBE), or with someone who was consciously trying to communicate with the person who witnessed his/her apparition."
- Parapsychologylab.com

197

Here again the OOBE is connected to BL, which is also freely interchanged with the word "apparition." Yet the word "apparition" is more closely interchanged with the word "ghost" or "spirit" or "entity," all of which give a different idea than what bilocation actually is. The terminology is frequently used mixed with some schools of remote viewing; please remember that words are important (this from a writer who has to use "spell check" repeatedly!) and that we should keep this in mind when reading articles about it. I have also seen "solid astral body" and "<u>bio</u>location" used as terms in place of BL. The writer might be meaning any number of these other things, which would result in further confusion of an already maligned and wondrous event.

Please get in the habit of respecting and using the right term for the right experience; this will help lend unity to the research and stories as they are compiled, and help everyone in keeping track and finding them. You don't have to use "BL," I just couldn't find an abbreviation anywhere that was being used for it. But, I think the word "bilocation" is the most popular term being used by the general public for someone physically seen in two or more places at once.

Bilocation a Pertinent Doctrine of the Catholic Church

"A mixed mode of location is that of a being circumscriptively in one place and definitely elsewhere, as is Christ in heaven and in the Sacred Host. This latter mode of bilocation is pertinent to the Catholic doctrine of the Holy Eucharist. All the physical laws of matter known to natural science contradict the bilocation of a material body as physically possible. As an absolute or metaphysical impossibility involving an intrinsic, essential contradiction, Catholic philosophers maintain that there is no intrinsic repugnance to a mixed mode of location. Since local extension is not an essential note of material substance, but merely a relation, bilocation does not involve the multiplication of a body's substance but only the multiplication of its local relations to other bodies." - New Catholic Dictionary

Next we have a belief of an inanimate object being also physically the flesh of

Jesus at some point of the Holy Eucharist service. All Christian churches that I know of celebrate Communion in some manner, although not all hold to this same bilocation tenant of faith with the Host. But, as we remember the mighty Padre electron, who can say - and if faith is added, and the Power is plugged in, we know anything can happen. On this note, please remember how many Catholic Saints and Fathers are known to have bilocation included with their other Supernatural gifts of levitation, healing miracles, etc.

"A mixed mode of location would be that of a being which is circumscriptively in one place (as is Christ in heaven), and definitively (sacramentally) elsewhere (as is Christ in the consecrated Host)...Being a resultant or quasi effect of quantity it may be suspended in its actualization; at least such suspension involves no absolute impossibility and may therefore be effected by Omnipotent agency. Should, therefore, God choose to deprive a body of its extensional relation to its place and thus, so to speak, delocalize the material substance, the latter would be quasi spiritualized and would thus, besides its natural circumscriptive location, be capable of receiving definitive and consequently multiple location; for in this case the obstacle to bilocation, viz., actual local extension, would have been removed." - New Advent Catholic Encyclopedia: Bilocation

Personal Research Results

On the DH research questionnaire, perhaps #52 holds the most opportunity for a client to answer if they experienced a bilocation event during the healing: *Did you wake up during the DH?* YES (52%) NO (40%) If so, please continue: *(listed by category, clients were asked to mark all that applied.* I felt a tingling sensation (72%) I felt a warm sensation (70%) I felt I was not alone (63%) I was not aware of any unusual feeling when I woke up (21%) Saw an image of the healer in the room (18%) Saw a mist, apparition, or image in the room (17%) saw an image of Christ, Angels, or other religious figure in the room (8%) Did any of these images appear as solid (NO 88%) YES (12%) hear any unusual sounds (12%) smell any unusual odors (10%) Other: (14%) *NOTE: "Other" included light in the room; disembodied arms or hands or face working over the body; seeing colors; hot sensations; animals acting strangely and waking the client up; and details of "unusual sounds" or "smells" (i.e. roses, chimes) etc.*

Some are self-explanatory, others let's take a closer look at: *"saw a mist, apparition, or image in the room"* may or may not be bilocation. *"Saw an image of Christ, Angels, or other religious figures in the room"* may or may not be bilocation (remember my first validated BL experience? The gentleman thought I was an Angel). The 18% that said *"I saw an image of the healer in the room"* may or may not be bilocation, but is the most intriguing, since the form was detailed enough to be recognizable as me. *"Hear unusual sounds"* (12%) only leads to further speculation, and may or may not be related to bilocation. But, if a person needs physical vocal cords to create an externally audio sound wave for a physical ear to receive (different from "clairaudience," where internal hearing occurs), perhaps a somewhat or fully physically manifested bilocation has occurred for a person to be able to write in their notes: *"someone called my name."*

This would have to correspond to the bilocater's desire for contact, and actually calling the client's name. In my case, I often speak to the person and say out loud prayers while I am being facilitated to heal them, so there is a possibility they could hear their name or other things that I am saying. It is interesting to note that 12% thought the images they saw were solid, and this may be some of the most convincing evidence of all, along with your own experience, of course.

Why Does Bilocation Occur?

I have noticed that only a few healings occur when I am in the RV phase, and being in full OOBE is where most of my distant healing time occurs and is the most beneficial. I have been greatly encouraged to see that the blessing of BL has the added benefit of wonderful healings, physically, emotionally and spiritually. I stand amazed at the outpouring and Oneness of Father's Love!

For I am not anyone special, only my Free Will choice was, to be used as a tool for a loving and compassionate Dad. I am grateful for whatever journey He takes me on, and sometimes it's a wild ride! But if we place *love* where fear lived, and *hope* where desperation wept, our enlightenment will

200

proportionately light stars where only dark embers were before. And you, dear one, will shine brightly and be brought into many darkened rooms because of the strength of your glow, and the shadows will disappear from before your face and those around you. You will manifest glory. Shine on!

"It's not about ability, nor inability, but availability..." - Traditional

St. Anthony of Padua

In 1227, St. Anthony of Padua, a Portuguese Franciscan friar, was in Limoges, France on Holy Thursday giving a sermon. During the sermon, he remembered that he was obliged to be chanting prayers with his fellow friars in their chapel across town. Realizing this, he stopped his sermon, knelt on the spot, pulled his hood over his head and became quite still. At that moment, Friar Anthony appeared in the chapel and chanted the prayers as required. When they were done, he simultaneously withdrew from the chapel and raised his head at the church - and continued with his sermon. - Paranormal.about.com

Sir Gilbert Parker

In 1905, Sir Gilbert Parker, a member of the British Parliament, was attending a debate in the House of Commons. During the debate, he noted that Sir Frederick Carne Rasch was also present, sitting in his usual spot. Yet this was impossible since Sir Frederick was quite ill with flu and, according to members of his household, remained in bed throughout the day. Apparently, Rasch's double was determined to hear the debate. - ibid

Padre Pio

Definitely the most well-known and documented bilocationist has been St. Padre Pio of Pietrelcina, Italy. Numerous books and articles have been written on his many gifts of healing, levitation, precognition, bilocation and numerous other chasms, and he is a more modern personage (d. 1968, canonized 2002) than many. Since so much information abounds, I will only cite a couple of small stories here; although I would suggest that further research into this adept will encourage and benefit the reader with how much *good* can come from BL.

"One day, a former Italian Army Officer entered the sacristy and watching Padre Pio said; "Yes, here he is! I am not wrong!" He approached Padre Pio, and kneeling in front of him crying, he said; "Padre, thank you for saving me from death." Afterwards, the man told the people present there, "I was a Captain of the Infantry and one day on the battlefield in a terrible hour of battle, not far from me I saw a friar who said; 'Sir, go away from that place!' I went towards him and as soon as I moved, a grenade burst in the place where I was before and opened a chasm. I turned around in order to find the friar, but he was not there anymore." Padre Pio, who was bilocating, had saved his life."

"A woman was at her daughter's home in Bologna. She had a tumor in her arm. So she agreed with her daughter to go for surgery. The surgeon told her to be patient and to wait some days before establishing a date for the surgery. In the meanwhile, her son-in-law sent a telegram to Padre Pio asking him to pray for his mother-in-law. At the moment when the telegram reached Padre Pio, the woman, who was in the dining room alone, saw a capuchin friar enter through the door. "I am Padre Pio of Pietrelcina," he said. Then, after asking her what the doctor had said and encouraging her to trust in Our Blessed Mother, he made the sign of the Cross on her arm and went out of the room. At that point, the woman called for the maid, her daughter and son-in-law. She asked them why they allowed Padre Pio to enter without announcing him. They responded that they had not seen Padre Pio and furthermore, they had not opened the door to anyone. The next day, the surgeon did a medical check-up on the woman in preparation for surgery; however, he could not find any tumor." - Catholicwebservices.com

Alex Tanous

"A man named Auerbach tells of a similar story of Alex Tanous, who is said to have bilocated to Canada while his body was seen by witnesses, slumped in a chair in New York. And the time of the events, Tanous was waiting to head out to a late lecture. His agent and at least one other person were with them when he sat down to rest. After Tanous closed his eyes in New York, his body

apparently showed up on a friend's doorstep in Canada. Tanous drank tea and chatted for a while before leaving. When the friend did not hear a car start, he looked out, worried that Tanous was stranded. He saw no tracks in the snow and no car. His wife, however, who was upstairs at the time, remembered hearing the conversation between Tanous and her husband. Also, it was noted that the dog started barking when Tanous first came to the door and reacted to his presence in the house. When Tanous straighten in his chair in New York, he told the people there that he had been to Canada and what had happened - all of which was later confirmed by the man and his wife in Canada." - The PK Zone by Pamela Rae Heath MD

Dr. Mark McDonnell

"Dr. Mark McDonnell a member of the British House of Commons, was laid up at his home in very ill when an important bill came before the house for a vote. McDonnell's solid Astro double was seen by dozens of witnesses to be debating this bill in the house for two days. His vote is on record, although there other witnesses proving that he never left his house during those two days." - The Unexplained by Allen Spraggett

Bilocation is Folding Space and Time

Perhaps the best description I have found for helping the analytical mind understand the "Big Three" of RV, OOB & BL is the explanation that David Morehouse gives about folding space. Although he is evidently referring to remote viewing when he talks about bilocation, I think the concept is probably the same:

"It's folding space, folding time and space. It's like bringing the event to you without ever going to the event, if you tap into it. It's omnipresent while traversing back and forth on the time-space continuum. What does it mean? It means you're everywhere at the same time. So the only way you can be everywhere at the same time is because everywhere is where you are. So folding space is the best analogy I can think of it like an accordion that folds in on itself, where you don't move. I was taught to believe that it was like the pages of a book, of an encyclopedia. There are planes that are separated, yet

203

they're connected by the spine of the book. The spine of the book corresponds to the unconscious. The biophysical body can travel in its own quantum reality, in effect tunneling through space-time. The physical body can be at one end of this quantum-reality wormhole, while the biophysical field is at the target site at the other end. When bilocation occurs, this quantum-reality wormhole is created." - David Morehouse, interviewed by Uri Dowbenko, for the article, *The True Adventures of a Psychic Spy*, in Nexus Vol 4 No 5, Sep 1997

Five Logical Steps for Bilocation

As I have stated before, dramatic power *beyond your own* is needed - and you probably won't know until it happens, if you are going to experience bilocation or not. But, without your own Free Will desiring to turn on the light switch, nothing is ever going to happen in the first place.

(1). Going from RV to an OOB to a BL is one logical route. When you are first in a 50/50 consciousness split (with RV), you become very familiar to everything around you, and the "logicalness" of where you are. You are incorporating the brain, and perhaps everything becomes "more real" this way, instead of going straight to OOB. You need to see the BL *as very real* for it to occur by your intention, instead of only spontaneously. I have also found it beneficial to hold an object related to my focus for an intentional BL - a picture of the person, place, map, physical item (i.e., a souvenir from the area), as a "touch-stone" to connection. *Always* start with prayer.

(2). After getting the logical information you desire through RV, let go of any writing apparatuses, stop talking, and let yourself "click out" for an OOBE. Now you will feel movement and "going" there, since your consciousness is actually not in your physical body any more. When you get there, it is a good idea to remind yourself for the reason you are there, since (at least in my case) fun and just looking around can be a big distraction! Say, for example, *"I am here to heal Elizabeth"* or *"Heal Elizabeth now."* Say what you need to for clarifying any normal OOBE, such as *"clarity now"* if things are foggy. Use the tool of time, decree it *now!*

(3). Now, with an intentional BL, get your astral body into position as close to being human as possible. For example, if you are horizontal, come upright and place your feet on the real floor or ground. This is difficult, since you can't feel any pressure at first in your out-bound body, and depending on how much you are able to manifest, gravity may do very little against any mass you first have. Hopefully, you have made your intention known beforehand, and now you wait on The Big Guy to see if BL will happen.

(4). When I arrive at the destination for the BL, I always find myself not fully where I need to be - God seems to choose the body's *formation* or manifestation out of sight, then I have a short distance to walk to where I need to be. I also leave quietly without notice, and so far no one has ever reported me just fading away. I have also found that time is very close to normal when you are in this state.

(5). Be discreet and humble, or it may not happen again. It may be just the sight of you is all that is needed (perhaps a comforting vision at a death-bed), and there is no need to manifest any longer than is necessary. The Big Guy takes care of all that. Wait if you keep feeling spacey. If you can't travel just by intention, but have to move your feet, that is a good sign you are actually manifesting. I try to pay real attention to the weight/gravity to let me know what is going on, but in my excitement, I have learned it is just easier to try the door handles first, instead of trying to go through them or walls, as in an OOBE. You'll find all this out on your own, sometimes the hard way, as you smack your face on something!

There is nothing to fear about "getting stuck" or manifesting with a chair in the middle of you, or between walls or something odd like that. Just stick to the plan and do what you need to do - remember The Big Guy is in charge of this stuff. If you want to go have fun, go on your own time and just have an OOBE. If you are doing this to prove something to yourself or to show off, you won't be successful in it. That is like using precognition in Vegas. It's not for the right reasons and wouldn't be blessed.

Developing Deeper Focus

Practice this at home. In your very quiet meditative space, just before you get to the opportunity to "click out," look at a flower in front of you (we are choosing something alive but still, about 18 – 24 inches from you). Really know that flower with all five senses. Truly *see* it, how the translucent petals delicately reflect the pastel shades. If this flower had a voice, or a song, what would it *sound* like? Make a choice in your head and hear this flower song. Whether it has a scent of its own or not, what *scent* do you attribute to this flower? What *flavor* would this flower leave on your tongue? If you *touched* this flower to your cheek, what would it feel like?

Now, *transfer your consciousness to this flower.* Go out of body, and become the flower, and come back again. Do these practices in short intervals, so that you remember everything when you return. Write down your adventure. In time, this will truly broaden your horizon, to how we are so very connected in the web of life. Whether it is a tree, or even an inanimate object such as a stone or a babbling brook, feeling the essence is incredible. *I have seen through the eyes of an eagle.* I have felt what he felt! Animals will (most of the time) be OK with this. The slower or larger the brain, the easier it is to ask -and get a response - unless there is food or sex around, which drowns out any request or ability for them to hear you. At that time, they don't respond at all, they have more important things on their mind!

I know what it feels like to be tiny, wet and curled up in a dark musty tunnel, with my belly full of skunk milk lying near mom and my brothers and sisters. This will expand your mind beyond any ego. I do *not* feel this is what the Native Americans and some other cultures call "shape-shifting." I am only borrowing the space, and not creating a separate one. I am simply asking permission of the life already there, to visit and interact for a limited time.

I have thought about this a lot, as to why we can do this, even for play. I think God allows it for only one reason - so we know the balance of the web of life, and how precious His works are, and to treat everything better - to truly KNOW we all shimmer together, in this glorious sea of our light connection. We are all in this together, and are in the Oneness. Have fun!
!
"So we fix our eyes not on what is seen, but on what is unseen. For what is

seen is temporary, but what is unseen is eternal." (2 Cor. 4:18)

CHAPTER 13
When Intention is Evil –
Transforming Negative Energy
Friends in High Places and Protection from Fallen Angels

"...it is a great encouragement to see that things which we thought impossible are possible to others, and how easily these others do them. It makes us feel that we may emulate their flights and venture to fly ourselves..." - Interior Castle by Teresa of Avila (16th century)

When negative energy is transformed by being filtered through the system of a highly realized being, enormous power is released. And the ripple effect is boundless. This is why there is no need to fear anything that you may come across; because you remember who you are and know that you are a child of the Light of God. This information applies whether you are out of the body or in. You are the one who chooses to stop the gossip instead of adding to it and passing it on - you are the one who takes the initiative to reach out to the homeless, the helpless, the poor and the sick. You are the one who uses what gifts you have been given to gift others, whether it is in a material way or the precious ingenuities of your spirit. However, if you do NOT have these qualities in your heart, you may get yourself into trouble and not recognize the life-line that has been thrown to you, and the results could be hazardous.

The Cry for Help versus the Transfer of Responsibility

There is a big difference between a cry for help and a transfer of responsibility. Those who cry out for Father's help will be Divinely led to the opportunity, information, teacher or some opportunity for receiving healing. But those who want to cling to their problems will not see the doors open to them, nor recognize any guidance from the other side. If these people come to me needing healing in any of the aspects of physical, emotional or spiritual health, my hands will only be warm, or even stay cold, since they are allowing very little or no healing into their "bubble" of Free Will.

At a soul level people can choose to believe and let all kinds of misinformation into their psyche by fear. For example, for the unhealthy person, perhaps their disease is the first time they have felt a support system and love of friends and family around them; and they think if they get well, they would lose this. Or, perhaps there is fear of healing because of loss of the guarantee of a monthly disability check. So we can see that Free Will can be ignored, or misused every day. We can choose to focus on the fear, instead of the love. We can make things out to be much bigger and more dramatic than they would really pan out to be. The whole thing is very simple – our choices are either Love or fear. We have the ability while still in these bodies to attune to the Infinite, ourselves, and to each other, all without fear, in the fullness of love. Think of what "attuned" means – one vibration resonating with and coming to a vibration of another. Which vibration do you attune with? Love or fear?

As the saying goes, *"there are no atheists on a sinking ship."* We sail under our own power; we decide we don't need to listen to the weather report; and the storm comes and overtakes us. We can stay there in a victim mentality and blame the wind and sea (and God) for swamping the vessel. Or, even at this late stage we can help ourselves by signaling the cargo ship close by, and turn on the bilge pumps the ship was originally built with and stay afloat and live. In other words, we have the choice to blame everyone and everything else for our troubles that we got ourselves into to begin with, and ignore any helpful opportunities that come by. Or we can ask for help while taking action ourselves. Or better yet, be receptive enough to observe, listen and pay attention to any signs beforehand and take corrective action.

Too many times people accept life's tragedies as "an act of God." They don't expect Him to change the inequalities of life, which makes religion only a method of acceptance of life's inadequacies. This is another inaccuracy, and a transfer of responsibility instead of a cry for help. People who accept this as true *will make it true* in their lives; they will experience and allow tragedy after tragedy without seeing a way out, *because they don't expect one.* They see themselves only as a victim, and that is that. But we do each have a choice.

The same holds true if you feel you are going to "get in trouble" while out of body. If you feel that you are going to be torn apart by terrible manifestations and demons, you will. That is the weakness and vibration that attracts those things to you, your fear and doubt of who you are as a child of God is like putting blood in the water for sharks. If you understand that you will see things that are negative, but it won't matter because they can't do anything to you because you are enveloped by God's Love, then that is what will happen. You protect yourself by the prayers, intentions and the expectations you have before your OOBE. If you ask for guidance and protection from the Holy Angels before you go, there is nothing to fear. And what is reflected in this very popular Psalm, *"though I walk through the valley of the shadow of death, I will fear no evil, for you are with me…"* (Ps. 23:1-6) Please realize you will see wondrous things as well!

Seeing the other side is a useful, interesting, and empowering thing. And fear of the other side and what might be seen is succumbing to fear and stagnation, and a victim mentality. This chapter will help you with some methods of protection from the darkness, and help you to come to a place of peaceful manifestation with prayer.

"That we can have these other reality experiences with our physical brains indicates they were designed to do so. We were meant to break out of this physical reality into a larger perspective. If these experiences are truly transformative, they will be dangerous to your old self, the part that doesn't believe in other worlds, realities, or forms of consciousness. So beware, transformation often comes after we move through the fear and the loss of self. We can deny that these other realities exist, but we can't stop experiencing them. They are a vital aspect of who we are."- Close Encounters of the Nightmare Kind by Patrick Marsolek

Prayerful Intentions and Manifesting Positive Influence

"Tiffany described a woman/spirit to me that God wanted her to tell me about. The woman described was my mother, down to the very last detail! My mom wanted me to know she had seen everything I had done in my life…was proud of me…thought my new house was beautiful! Years of emotion and pain were released, as I realized Mom's love for me, and God's. I had felt so

alone, and angry that she had not been part of my life - now I know she has always been there. Even though she died when I was only eight." - J.S. Australia

"Dear Tiffany, Thank you sooo much for the divine healing last night. It was very uplifting what came through…also, I felt it when it happened, and my whole body was warm. I actually thought I saw you there in the room. I woke up dreaming about my mother. When you emailed me the results, and you had a message from mom, I knew it wasn't a dream! I have your notes and what she said on my dresser so I can see it every day…Also, the fibroid tumors do not hurt anymore…the arthritis is much better…I actually feel lighter and younger, I look for the healing to continue. I thank our Father for you…Love, B.T." Colorado

"Tiffany, just a note, to tell you thanks. I never expected the healing to work, and I can tell you my shoulder is now fully mobile and pain-free. And even when you described my father, down to the last detail, and how he died, I was skeptical. But when you saw him and I re-building lawn mowers and bicycles together, I knew my dad was really there. I hadn't cried about his death until then. I am going to contact my mom and tell her to get that test done that you suggested (that DAD) suggested, and tell her about what happened, whether she believes me or not. I am a believer. People don't really die. Miracles happen. God Bless - A.M." California

You Have Friends in High Places

One of the most exciting and amazing experiences a person can have is a conscious meeting with a loved one who has transitioned in death. It gives us comfort in many ways: it proves without a doubt that we live on beyond the physical body; and that we never have to lose contact with those who have died.

"…interactions with conscious entities seem to be happening…Based on personal experience they seem to be a natural byproduct of playing with remote viewing and the paranormal." – Remote Viewing Secrets by Jospeh McMoneagle

There have always been stories of loved ones contacting their family and friends through supernatural means. One study reports that *more than two-thirds* of all people have had the experience of seeing an apparition of a deceased loved one (*Spiritual Healing: Scientific Validation of a Healing Revolution* by Daniel J. Benor M.D.). Remote viewing, near-death experiences and the out of body experience are some of these supernatural touchstones that allow this communication. Often, interaction or awareness of the other side is a by-product of distant healing.

The Differences between Spirits and Ghosts

In an OOB state, we learn first-hand that our consciousness can exist very well outside of our human form. We then understand beyond a doubt, that when a person physically dies, the vibratory rates change, but the essence of the person is still very much alive and conscious. This is why it's so common for us to be visited, *because they can!* One of the main reasons people have initially tried OOB is to consciously communicate with their dead loved ones. *Many have been successful,* and return with the calmness of knowing they have not been separated from each other, and that their loved ones live on as *spirits.* Spirits are very bright, and will often appear "physically" similar to how you remember them, so they will be recognizable to you. But left on their own, they normally appear around 30 years of age, a typical time of top physical maturity and vitality on earth, which they like to remember and imitate.

Please keep in mind that departed loved ones who have gone to the Light are still *not* in charge of your life issues. When it comes to *your* stuff, you have your own decisions to make because you came in with your own tasks for this journey. They have released all their ego and old stuff, and because of this, they are much kinder and easier to get along with than they were in real life. But, with everything they tell you, you still need to check it out for yourself, since it has to ring true with the voice inside of you for what is best for you and your situation. They are not God. Each of us is in a different place in our lesson book, and clarity on one issue may not mean clarity on another, since during our lives we are all working on different facets of love.

213

But, spirits do have access to Divine knowledge and are sometimes utilized in an Angel capacity, to be a "messenger" to tell you something. So listen to what they have to say, just remembering it has to feel right and make sense to you. Also, there is the very real danger of a dark spirit masquerading as your loved one, when they are not. Fallen Angels manipulate very actively and easily, they have lived for a very long time and know the full details of your loved one intimately, because they see their life unfold, as well as yours. So the utmost of precautions must be in place to not fall prey to the emotions you may feel when first contacted by a deceased person. Put them through their paces first. There are cosmic laws in place regarding this ploy, and these Angels know they are going "against the law."

So, the easiest way to figure out who is who, is to call the "police" on them, for example, asking the manifestation to say "I love Jesus now" is a quick and easy way to sort it all out. Why use a personal name, why Jesus? Do not ask it to say "I love God," since God is a title and not a name, and they can say they love God and be recognizing an entirely different entity than who you're thinking about. If it is a demon, it cannot say that they love Jesus now, and will disappear, curse or try to change the subject. Then you know. It really is that simple. Whether you are a Christian or not, this works, since the demons all know who is who, and how Dad feels about Him, and the warrior position He has now. Best way to irritate the Father is to mess with the son! And we put the word *now* in, because many *did* love the son before they rebelled with their Free Will. So asking how they feel *now* is key to which side they are on *at this time*.

"You believe there is one God. Good! Even the demons believe that – and shudder." (Js 2:16)

After a person dies, there is a "debriefing" that occurs for 2-3 weeks, where full understanding of that person's life course is realized. But, that person still does not have all understanding of *your* life course; and it is not his purpose to do so. So looking for loved ones to answer *our* questions and guide *our* lives is neither wise nor necessary. Simply acknowledging them, giving them love, appreciation and respect is all they need; and you receiving theirs. They want

214

to see you happy, tell you *"I love you"* and that they know what you are doing and are proud of you. You have not lost them. Any suggestions they make along the way are only from their own perceptions to help you - unless it is a message from God, and then it is a whole different thing. All along the way, you must still accept the consequences for your choices, as you are a creature of Free Will.

Ghosts – What Purgatory Really Is

Ghosts were humans that died but have not yet gone to the Light of Divine Love, and thus have not experienced their life review or a debriefing time. Ghosts are folks with unfinished business to do here and won't let it go, or they fear they don't deserve to go to God, so their own fear prevents them from doing so. They equate the Death Angel (the word "Homing Angel" actually fits better, since he is a very maternal and wonderful Spirit) with a place of pain and suffering (hellfire is another manipulation of misinformed religion), or they just haven't accepted that they truly are dead.

Sudden death is more apt to bring this difficulty up. Ghosts have a lower vibration than spirits do, and are easier to see, even to the point of detailed facial features. They also are worried and anxious, and sometimes outright mean. This place of being "in-between" is where the real idea of purgatory came from. And yes, it is appropriate to pray for those in this personal place of struggle, that they made open to Love; just as it is appropriate to keep in our prayers any person in difficulty, alive or dead.

In all deaths, when the Homing Angel appears, they come with spirits of loved ones, relatives, friends and even pets. This helps encourage the departed that this is real and not an illusion, since the person may think this is a dream and not the reality. If they do not go with the Angel (since Free Will is always in place), they end up in a *holding pattern* repeating many strong memories and actions over and over again, instead of going with the Angel and their loved ones to God.

This is where "haunting" comes in, and the need for some of us who can see both sides, or to see them during OOBE or RV, to help these to be aware of

215

their situation, see the difference between fact and fiction, and help point them home. Ghosts are the easiest to see of all the categories, since their low vibration give them a density that higher vibrations do not. Do not listen to what ghosts have to say, since they speak out of fear, guilt, anger and stagnation. You need to be the one speaking to them, to help them along if you choose to do this. Neither ghosts nor spirits show up with injuries on them, unless they want to show you for verification purposes who they are, how they died, or if the ghost identifies very strongly with the injury or deformity and cannot move past it.

Sometimes, ghosts will constantly repeat how they died, or the most traumatic scenes of their lives, because they literally can't see anything past that, and the trauma has clogged up memories of other things. You will see the scenes also, since their consciousness is powering an energy-tracing of their memory. These can be traumatic to view, but now you know why you see them, and are nothing to fear. It is simply another tool you can use to help them make new decisions and be on their way. Do not be overly upset if a ghost will still not move on, since Father will continue to give them new opportunities to change their minds and blend into the peace and unity that eagerly awaits them. He cares for every one of us, but will not force the issues. How wonderful when we accept how much we are loved while we are still in the body and living – this makes for such less confusion for us and an easier transition too.

Various Unidentified Life-forms and UFOs

"Many are unaware that during sleep we move slightly out of sync with our biological bodies. This provides a potential window of direct communication with our minds...Those who are trained and comfortable with out-of-body exploration possess an enormous advantage because their consciousness is far more open and prepared for this multidimensional contact and communication. In other words, they are far more likely to experience spiritual visitations in full awareness." – The Secret of the Soul by William Buhlman

Many people report out of body experiences where they astrally meet with a teacher or guide, someone whom they do not recognize from earth. I have seen a great variety of beings in all different shapes and sizes, and many are simply variations of Angels in various forms in capacities fulfilling what work they need to do, and in the bodily form they were created to do it in.

I have been told there are many visitors which are only allowed to *observe* and *not interact* with the world in any way. We are in "containment" right now, and onlookers view us similar to how we may view animals in a zoo. This containment is because of the Original Issues that were raised here upon the earth about God's right to rule. Until this *court case* of evidence is satisfied and the case is closed, there will be no interaction beyond those who were here when the case started. Any UFO interaction with humans that has been blamed on "extraterrestrials" has simply been Fallen Angels mimicking and manipulating situations to blame on these other life forms and Holy Angels. This is the same thing theses demons do when they sometimes appear as deceased loved ones or "Angels of Light." Discernment is needed in all things, and protection put in place before you judge who and what you interact with.

Since I rely so heavily upon Father's words and empirical evidence, I am careful to shield my conclusions from anything I have read or might piece together analytically in my head. I do the same with the crime scene investigations. You will never catch me watching a TV show about murders, missing children, etc. I don't want to construct a hidden "memory" that subconsciously might be tapped into and muddy an investigation. I don't want to THINK I know something, I want to KNOW I know something. *There is a big difference.* And what you put *in the computer* of the brain, is what you get out of it. So, I choose to let the computer download new programs that are virus-free from the Eternal Programmer, and do not use "share-ware" for this kind of important information gathering.

Some of the beings and life-forms will acknowledge your presence in the out of body state, but don't seek them out to help you. Only call upon Father and those He would send, which may be the Holy Angels or even ascended masters to help you. I find it interesting most other life-forms don't want to acknowledge their individual awareness of you. I have wondered if they cannot recognize the difference between our sleeping astral projection, or a conscious one. Or, perhaps this makes no difference to them, and they are simply very aware of the limited-interaction rule in force for the moment. For example, the interaction could be likened to starfish, fish, dolphins and a myriad of sea creatures in the great ocean (these various spiritual beings), and we are just the plankton floating by. There doesn't really seem to be any real attention being paid to us. Everyone has their own thing to do, and it is all very important to them. The fact that we may be aware while in our OOB state seems to mean little to them, if it is recognized at all; and this prevents any potential problems from occurring.

Ascended Masters on Earth

The most interesting connections are with folk still here on earth who have come in with a high place of awareness and enlightenment, *during* their time in the human physical body. Most of the time these "ascended masters" are still choosing to interact and influence people with simple invisible or spiritual proddings, much like the Angels do. They are most helpful on both sides - whether in the body or out of it - so you may find them on the other side in your travels. I have found that *ascended* doesn't necessarily mean you are dead! All of the masters I have met on the astral plane still have kept a human form, and are very bright and loving. All of them had a choice to come back or not – they had finished polishing their facets of love and did not *need* to come back to complete anything more. But, they have chosen to anyway, to help during this special time on earth. Some of these ascended masters you may know in their physical body right now, and often exist as a child of mankind in bodies that are considered "not normal" by society's standards, by having Downs, or numerous other differences that allow them to barely be *in* the body while highly functioning well beyond it.

Each spirit of these special people also has *another color mixed into the brightness.* They remind me of *low wattage* Holy Angels. On the astral plane it is as if the fish is back in the water, and they are tranquil, beautiful and friendly, and always ready and willing to teach, help and share. Gone is any frustration felt while they are in the body. And in your astral journeys, if these fully enlightened souls cannot help you at the moment, they will introduce you

218

to someone who can. One ascended master/teacher can help numerous humans, and the earth as well, and they treasure this opportunity to do so, since they know the power and ripple effect of intention with the Greatest Master of all, and are vessels to Love's expansion.

All masters know each other very well, and they know who's still on the planet, and who's not. They are one of the best links between God and humans in many situations, since they understand the nuances of how we experience and feel things. They intervene and interchange communication freely with the Angels. They are patient and kind, and take the roles of guide and teacher interchangeably as needed: a teacher teaches; a guide encourages growth in what was taught. A master knows what is needed at any given time for the progress of the spiritual essence, they are in full Connection.

Spiritual Guides

You may have different spiritual guides interact with you at different times, depending on what you need and their experience to help you, and different masters, but all acknowledge the One Greater than themselves, and their oneness with you. They also interact freely with you while you are *in* the body, and may stay with your physical body while you are *out*.

Guides seem to be a connection between the color each one has mixed in their glow and the emotion they most exude and teach. This was a revelation to me! And now it makes sense to me why one guide will go and another come in as we advance. They each have their own specialties. They also seem to multi-locate on the spiritual plane, as I have seen the same one in several places, talking with different souls, in quick relation to each other. But I know it is also possible that they might have just moved quickly from one place to another where I happened to be. So, I see no reason why they *wouldn't* multi-locate, as it would seem to benefit them as an aid in taking care of the heavy responsibilities they have in helping so many, as being a touch-stone to The Big Guy.

All masters encourage independence and growth toward the Cosmic Heart, and not dependence or codependence on them or their teachings. They are here to help you remember who *you* are.

Messages from Angels, Influences of Demons

You can always spot the Angels! They have such a high vibration, that even while in the OOB state, they are magnificently brilliant and their individual facial features cannot be clearly seen because of the haze of glow. For years I could only see them by *raising* my own vibration extremely high, and they choosing to *lower* theirs - and then perhaps a fleeting glimpse could be seen. But, now it is easier since the brightening that has come with the regeneration of stigmata, so I get to see them all the time! For you, it may be much easier to see them while you are out of body: they sparkle white and gold, and shimmer with iridescent rainbow colors. They come in all sizes and shapes, responsibilities and ranks, and all were all created for specific duties. Some are huge, over 40 feet tall, and some are minutely small. All are vessels of Love.

Some are "go-betweens" to deliver messages between Spirit and human (both the Greek *ag'ge-los* and Hebrew *mal-'akh'* actually mean *"spirit messenger"*). Angels are *not* humans who were once alive, and they all have Free Will. They were the first creations, the first sparks off the Divine Flame. The very *first* spark was called Michael the Archangel, who was later known by the name Jesus Christ and the "first-begotten son of God." Hence, another reason to "pull rank" on the demons by asking the question of them when discerning who around you is good or bad, since they were all brothers at one time, and they know Jesus and He knows them. And they know the rank and reward God gave Christ for the Love that was shown through fulfilling the responsibilities given; including His warrior status.

A bit more on what you might see and why, just to fill you in so you will not have fear. Here are more details to the story. Some Angels rebelled, and did their own thing outside of God-given responsibilities and chose for themselves what they felt was right and wrong, thus creating their own law. These rebellious ones are not utilized for Divine responsibilities any longer, but rather do the opposite - these *push* or influence people toward choices of fear and darkness, and the subsequent bad consequences of cause-and-effect. These negative influencers are called devils, demons, or Fallen Angels. They

220

try to manipulate behind the scenes. You might see them present themselves as deformed misty human figures (though they were never human), or as dark bat-like creatures with claws at the edge of their two sets of wings. Also, they can - most infamously - appear as an "Angel of Light," the thought of which instills fear into many people. There is no need for you to fear this, since you have the tools for discernment as given earlier.

If an Angel told you to jump off a cliff, or murder someone or take your own life, would you? Let's hope not - I have faith that you will know something is really "rotten in Denmark" if you act on these things! Father is big on Free Will, and specific prayerful intent. If you are *ever in doubt, pray it out,* and ask for validation from Father on your choices. You will receive back the answers you need, without having to guess. And it will *feel* right too, in your very essence.

There is a big court case going on right now needing the passage of time (thousands of years) for the evidence to pile up. We are in a speeding up of time because these issues are now at a close. This case is about Gods' authority to rule over what He has created, and His ability to make laws and reinforce them, which includes God's right to rule over mankind. Three Original Issues were brought up: (1). Man only loves God for what man can get out of God. (2) Man can guide himself successfully independent from God's Will (3) If a man is threatened with physical injury he will do anything to save himself, including cursing God to save his skin. You can see how this has played out through the rise of fall of all forms of governments in all parts of the world; how people throughout time have freely laid down their life for one another and for God; and how through struggle and difficulty people still love God. When closed, this court case will *never* have to be repeated in any other part of the grid of the cosmos ever again, since it has been settled here. Though it can be difficult, do you see how you are living in a part of history that you'll eagerly be talking about for timelessness to come? We get to witness and be a part of settling these Original Issues first-hand!

I am spending extra time with and giving you this information because it is important – and because you *will see* the Fallen Angels, you *will hear* the mocking and cursing, you may even *feel* the cold negative energy from their presence. But you must remember *they cannot do you any harm* unless you allow it. And you and Father will not allow it! Do not be afraid. Fear is the opposite of love, and will shut down any advancement you are making. Just know this: *it is not ever about attacking evil, but becoming brighter.* Love covers a multitude of darkness and protects you always. Even sending out the prayerful intentions of love against the demons is a wonderful idea, with positive cause-and-effect ripples coming back to you. That is how Love and Light is.

Can Anything Enter Into My Body When I Am Out of It?

No – nothing can enter your *home body* while you are clicked out. Nothing! Your body is on automatic, just like you are when sleeping at night, and you escape it every night, whether you remember it or not. Look for the "silver cord" attached from your physical body to your spirit body the next time you are OOB. Nothing can break this but death on the earth plane. Travel and have fun! Expand your awareness of this life, this earth, and one another. There are no limits unless you make them. Remember, there is no fear unless you allow it. Your Free Will of calling in alignment to Love protects you while you are out; and your guides protect and stay with your physical body.

In his classic book *Far Journeys,* Robert Monroe answers a question from a reader who was concerned about meeting a being while OOB: 'how can you tell if it is malevolent or benevolent?' *"...consciously limit your input "frequency," as it were, allowing only those on your "wavelength" to communicate and/or make contact with you. At best if there is a question, pat it on the shoulder and tell it to go home. At worst, you go back to the physical and regroup..."*

The One Place Where God Cannot Go – the Bubble of Free Will

For me to talk about God and for you to take any of it seriously, you have to know who and how I perceive this One to be, and then you need to hold it up to your essence and see if these things ring true to you or not. Never give your own power away. Always check things out first. I am answering not from the traditional religion I was taught, but by everything I have experienced and learned from the near-death experiences, stigmata, and every healing and OOBE I have had since then. *And still I am but a babe in the woods - I do not know it all!*

Though I am considered an authority in many of these things, I assure you that I am in a steady *continuum* of learning. The word "continuum" fits very well here, since it denotes a continuous seamless series, a link between two things, a continuous series of things that blend into each other so gradually and seamlessly that it is impossible to say where one becomes the next. For example, a rainbow is a *continuum* of color. And that is where I am, in a constant state of becoming, and remembering, and asking, and receiving. Then sharing what I am learning, which I hope encourages you to remember, ask, receive and share also! We are all in this together!

At the first NDE, when I stood in front of the bright light of His Divine Love, I knew that I was in front of the *physical center* of Source, of All Consciousness. I found God to be the source and reason for all things, but to also have *a central physical location of consciousness too.* He is *both* "out there," *and* "in here." There is a knowing of Oneness in all things, all things being part and particle of the One, that we feel deep inside our core. From my spirit body floating there in space, to the blade of grass back on earth, and every life-force in-between and beyond, the essence of God is felt and demonstrated everywhere. There is no separateness; no place that God is not…that is, *no place except one.*

An interesting thing…when I asked Father about Free Will, I saw what looked like the skin of a rubber balloon hanging around us. These were either inflated and bubbled out, or laid flat against the body and joined like a second skin. When it is inflated, there is definite *space around us* - a bubble of sorts - *this is the bubble of individual Free Will.* When a person "does their own thing," or uses their own Free Will, it creates opportunity for messing up, that is for sure, and it also creates a feeling of separation and desperate loneliness. Either way, it is the cause and effect of our own choices independent from God's Will. But, when we align our will with God's Will, the separation disappears, the bubble becomes "second skin," and we are plugged in and guided in the highest of endeavors, sort of like being on Divine cruise control. Then separation becomes simply an illusion for us, and we lead a blessed and abundant life. Father still asks for our input in what gives us the most joy and happiness – for this is the fulfilling of the purpose and true potential He created us to be – in loving Him, and our neighbor as ourselves. He joins with us to attain that goal – we choose our will to transform to His Will, but *it is not about sitting out the dance*. It is just about learning to follow the dance partner instead of being the one leading the steps.

It is the place in our journey of allowing and surrendering control to the one who knows how to drive the car, since in our imperfections and "drunkenness" at the moment, we are driving unsafely and could hurt ourselves or another unless we give up the keys. In that *not fully aware* state trying to drive and navigate on our own can lead to some tricky situations. In our stubbornness we insist we do not need any maps because we know exactly where we are, where we are going, and the best way to get there all on our own. Also, we often stubbornly refuse to do any maintenance on our car or open the instruction manual because it just might tell us that it is due for some work.

In fact, you may not have previously known it as a simple car owner, but even now as we speak there is a squabble going on with the powers that be because the question was brought up that a new car owner doesn't need his manual, that he is his own mechanic, and will figure it out even better on his own. This parallels the Original Issues from the Fallen Angels; paraphrased - that mankind can guide his own footsteps successfully without God, that man only loves God for what man can get out of God, and that man will trade his integrity to God to sustain his own life. Well, we've had thousands of years of history to show the results of that! *The car doesn't run!*

This simple story illustrates why we must consciously shift our awareness outside of ourselves and allow trust and faith to bridge the gap to Love, beyond our own control. Giving intention to prayer, we plug in to all that is of light and joy. Then we enlighten, and glow, and there is no feeling of separation any more. We are not "puffing" ourselves up with a false idea of protection, when actually we are causing separation. Choosing to align our will with His Will is what safely brings ourselves out of dead-end roads and impassable blocked ravines. Then, we don't feel separated, and everything starts to drive on "automatic" even on the sharpest of curves, and we get to kick back and enjoy the view!

Be Prepared to "See" Beyond Outward Appearances

Before, you saw only with the physical eyes of flesh, but here in this OOB world you experience new sight, including glimpses of darkness and demons, and beautiful bright beings, loved ones and Angels. And, as an added perk, if you "click out" in real-time, you will also be able to choose your physical companions more wisely than ever before. How? Because when you are in the altered astral state, you can ask to notice the spiritual brightness of people, and the oscillation of their vibrational state, *which corresponds to the facets of love they have been working on and the goodness of their soul.* What an inside track to choose our mates and friends! The spirit is shaped like a "golf tee" in the head and down the spine. You will see different shades of brightness in different people, they will glow brightly or be a variety of darkness or shadow. This is also an opportunity to be actively prayerful for those who are not as "bright" as they could be, asking for Love to be sent back to them and for them to recognize the Divine opportunities that open to them to know Love more fully. This is another beautiful perk of going out of body, to recognize another opportunity for encouraging love and connection and remembrance of each of us in our true, bright nature.

CHAPTER 14

The Path of the Mystic - Becoming True Potential
Becoming a Junction Point between Two Worlds

In a crowd, they look like everyone else. They are not going to appear the wealthiest, nor the most beautiful, nor the tallest or most popular, nor the slimmest. By looking at their outward appearance, the only recognizable difference may be the brightness of their eyes, their compassionate smile, or their welcoming but quiet nature. If you should decide to look for the mystic, you will find them everywhere; once you know what to look for.

There's one now - she is in the grocery store; the one that is never first in line, but places the old men and women with small children ahead of her. She is the one playing "peek-a-boo" with the baby in the neighbor's cart as she passes by, the one who makes a point to place an item back on the shelf that someone else dropped. She is the one who actually talks to the person in the wheelchair and asks if there is something they can get from the top shelf. There's another one – the guy at the gas station who could have gone first, but flagged you to go ahead. He's also the one who stopped in the rain to help change your flat tire. He's the one that makes sure you have enough helpers on moving day, pitches in, and then calls to make sure you made it to your destination.

You could still feel their presence long after you departed, and the thought of them brings a smile to your face and a twinkle to your eye. The surge of friendliness and hope you felt well up inside of you encouraged you to look for the splendor in all things. An oasis of peace bathed the time like an effervescent waterfall of golden bliss. You felt enlightened, loved, more connected to your heart, fully accepted, and true compassion for all other things. Anything was possible, attainable, and exactly available when and where they should be.

These Connectors are messengers of light, those whose very soul blazes unselfishly like a guiding torch throughout the night, one who lights the way through the darkness. This is not a person who USES healing, intuitive and psychic ability or unconditional love. This is a person who IS healing, intuitive and psychic ability and unconditional love. True enlightenment is not something you *do,* it is something that you *are,* and are constantly *becoming.* This mystic may be a friend, a spouse, a child, a father, or the person looking back from the mirror. This person may be *you!*

"...a mystic is not a special kind of human being, but every human being is a special kind of mystic." – Br. David Steindl-Rast

What is a Mystic?

I would like to ask you some personal questions, to help you honestly evaluate your life at this time. Are you happy? Do you have peace and tranquility in your life? Do you have a sense of purpose, and do you feel you are fulfilling it? Do you wake up each morning anticipating the joy and adventure of the day ahead? Do you feel secure about your future?

To know how far you have progressed, you need to know where you are right now. Do you have the courage to set your foot upon the path without knowing when you will get there, or what route it might take? Do you know why you stumble where you do, why you seem to go in circles sometimes, without forward momentum? Can you actually feel Presence upon your life and the warmth of personal guidance? All these questions are asked by the one yearning for the deeper things, and the desire to live life to the fullest. It is the life path of the *mystic.*

The word "mystic" is translated as *"someone who believes in the existence of realities beyond human comprehension,"* or *"one who has experience of union or direct communion with ultimate reality."* This is a person who acquires personal experience of the supernatural beyond human comprehension. In Christianity this experience usually takes the form of a vision or sense of union with Christ; however, there are also other forms of mysticism throughout the world.

The term *"mysticism,"* Greek, meaning *"to conceal."* In the Hellenistic world, *"mystical"* referred to *"secret"* religious rituals. - <u>Stanford Encyclopedia of Philosophy</u>. *"Mysticism"* generally being translated *as "a theory postulating the possibility of direct and intuitive acquisition of ineffable knowledge or power."* - Merriam-Webster Unabridged Dictionary. Although the word "mystic" may not be in common use now, at one time those devoted to spiritual paths were always considered mystics. Today, the term is sometimes used haphazardly by anyone who may wish to appear to have a link with the supernatural, but the true mystical heart of all ages is a humble one and desires not the praise of others but communion with ultimate reality itself.

"...It may also be accompanied by unusual experiences of ecstasy, levitation, visions, power to read human hearts, to heal, and to perform other unusual acts. Mysticism occurs in most, if not all, the religions of the world, although its importance within each varies greatly. The criteria and conditions for mystical experience vary depending on the tradition, but three attributes are found almost universally. First, the experience is immediate and overwhelming, divorced from the common experience of reality. Second, the experience or the knowledge imparted by it is felt to be self-authenticating, without need of further evidence or justification. Finally, it is held to be ineffable, its essence incapable of being expressed or understood outside the experience itself." - Joan A Range

Discovering the Hidden Universe

I know that Norway exists – I can tell you about the rocky fjords, the icy gray sea, the goats in the high country, and the ancient Viking ship on display at the Oslo museum. I have never been there, but I know it exists; along with all the relatives I've never met who make up my mother's ancestry. Perhaps I will visit one day, but I don't have to see it to know it is there. Does that boggle the imagination, or is that common sense? I can't see the wind either, but I can see the leaf blowing on the tree limb, and feel the breezes warm against my skin.

I am aware of the manifestations that signal wind's existence; and also gravity, microwaves, etc, even though they are all invisible to my eyes. And, I know and understand that I am subject to all the laws and interactions of these unseen forces of gravity, wind, microwaves, etc., even though I may not understand how they work.

Life-force energy (Holy Spirit) is of Divine Love and Intelligence (God) permeating all things through a cosmic vibrational language of Light (Christ). I *know* this exists, it is not a belief to me, it is a knowing. I don't have to believe in God; I *know* God. *Does that boggle the imagination, or is that common sense?* Ask your soul, see if it makes absolute sense and feels right. When the balloon of isolation is abandoned, and the static of chaos is removed, we become the pure stereo receivers we were hard-wired to be. *All of us* have the capacity to heal; to see things outside of physical eyesight; to manifest in places beyond our local space; to travel consciously through the dimensions of space and time. We are all in various states of *becoming.* We are all made in the image of God, becoming the true potential He created us to be.

The true goal of the mystic quest is not merely to understand and enjoy, and it is not just for the gifts. It's not even for happiness – all these things are added as the attainment is realized. There are no words to define how the soul's passion is fulfilled – it is pure union, total absorption, deified love. It is the passion of lovers in ecstasy, the full spectrum of the rainbow, and every voice in perfect harmony. It is not an end or suppression of any kind; but merely a beginning, an intensification of everything. Perhaps it can be likened to the quandary of the poets all through the centuries who have tried, in vain, to describe love. There are no human words to describe the face of God.

"...in the state of Divine Consciousness...the individual learns to transfer himself from a center of self-activity into an organ of revelation of universal being, and to live a life of affection for and one-ness with, the larger life outside...it is a gradual and complete change in the equilibrium of the self. It is a change whereby that self turns from the unreal world of sense in which it is normally immersed, first to apprehend, then to unite itself with Absolute Reality: finally, possessed by and wholly surrendered to this Transcendent Life, becomes a medium whereby the spiritual world is seen in a unique degree operating directly in the world of sense...no true mystic stays on the

mountain, but is known by the power beyond self to come down and change the world." – Mysticism by Evelyn Underhill

The Rhythm of the Cosmic Heart

In my own journey, people have often had the mistaken impression that I'm facilitated for miracles because of the lightning strike or the near-death experiences. *This is not the case – it was simply the tool used to awaken me!* We are *all* given defining moments in our lives, when the choices we make will advance our journey or not, and this was mine. When it came, I was given a choice – I just freely chose to surrender and accept the calling that was so graciously offered – I totally replaced my will with God's Will. I was the raindrop falling into the mighty ocean; when I surrendered my single identity, I found unity with everything. With this release, my ideas of isolation and separation (with its many accompanying negative and constricting concepts), was replaced with All-Encompassing Love and Light. At that very moment, while I was still out-of-body, a shift occurred, a much better "plugging in," if you will. I felt a child-like sense of wonderment as a warm flood of bliss and peace overcame me, and a warm tingling sensation filled me to my very toes.

As you have seen, it was at this time that I was told, *"Welcome to the world of healers,"* something I had never believed in before, since my background negated such things. As the experience continued, reams of information from that heavenly Community of Spirit flooded my being with sacred and wonderful things. As I fulfill the calling, by writing, speaking, teaching, healing, etc., the information flows effortlessly, and I hear myself saying and writing things that I never knew that I knew before! It is quite interesting for me, I am learning many things.

Especially since the stigmata began, my core essence is in a state of *constant entrainment,* a *becoming of resonance* that offers balance to others too. As one facilitated for healing miracles, I simply create an opportunity for others to hear the song the orchestra is playing. Perhaps there will be a recognition that you, too, have been one of the musicians all along, playing violin in the first string section. And *then,* you heal, *then* you become intuitive, etc., as a by-product of it all, because you have recognized who you are. So, how can I do these miraculous things? Because I am a child of God – just like you! We are the same. *Remember who you are and your true nature as a heartbeat in the pulse of God. We all dance to the rhythm of the Cosmic Heart, and that same beat pulses in your chest as well as mine.*

The Cosmic Heart is beyond time and expectation. Today's enlightenment may help you to understand history (including your own) and guide your future choices, but time is not a restriction on *becoming*. You have all the time in the world, yet every moment is precious! How you spend your time determines the value of *timelessness*. It is not about earning love, it is about giving it away. It is not about gaining material advantages, but you'll find that abundance will naturally come your direction as well. Your Holy intentions and high vibration of Light you are sharing with mankind will bring all the good things of the world to your feet. You won't need to be overly concerned with your needs next month or next year, because you *know* you will be taken care of.

To the average person, this may seem foolish. Others may see your dedication to the journey as a waste of time. But, you know who you are, and you won't be distracted or thrown off course by a rough wind. You simply wish the doom-and-gloom people well, send a prayer of love their way and go about your business. You realize that most people spend much of their lives in fear and repetition, while you have trimmed your sails and are drinking the cup of celestial nectar in your grand adventure on the high seas!

"To be able to integrate the various overlapping dimensions of consciousness in an ongoing trajectory is to struggle to be virtuous. Ensouled persons are on a quest to have the true, the good, and the beautiful coincide. They are in a process in which consciousness transcends itself. Mystics of all traditions maintain that, through meditation and other techniques, it is possible to silence all the patterns and operations of consciousness, to bring all the sensing, questioning, imagining, analyzing, and evaluating to a halt. What emerges from this cessation of activity, this emptiness, is a new kind of fullness, an awareness of what Meister Eckhart calls the Ground of Consciousness, and what other mystics have referred to variously as True Self, Great Mind, and God." – Geography of the Soul: An Intellectual Map

by S. Happel and J. Price

The Beautiful Water Crystal of Love and Gratitude

In his now-famous books, Dr. Emoto showed that high-speed photography of crystals formed in frozen water reveal definite changes when specific, concentrated thoughts are directed toward them. This is another quantum mechanic factor that we have seen with the changes that the act of observation made on random number generators (RNG). Through Dr. Emoto's photographs beautiful crystals emerge with good, harmonious and loving intentions; while misshaped ones emerge with bad, angry or polluted ones. When we remember that the human body is 70% water, it reminds us how important it is to only operate on and reflect positive vibes. So what creates the most beautiful and perfect crystal formed? Dr. Emoto writes:

"I particularly remember one photograph. It was the most beautiful and delicate crystal that I had so far seen – formed by being exposed to the words "Love and Gratitude." It was if the water had rejoiced and celebrated by creating a flower in bloom. It was so beautiful that I can say that it actually changed my life from that moment on. Water had taught me the delicacy of the human soul, and the impact that "love and gratitude" can have on the world...this is supposedly what all the world's religions are founded on, and if that were true, there would be no need for laws... "Love and Gratitude" are the words that must serve as the guide for the world."- The Hidden Messages in Water by Dr. Emoto.

Being thankful and in a constant state of gratitude immerses us in a wholeness of receiving perfect wholeness at all levels. Mystics don't have to tell The Big Guy what to do, because that gives power and focus to a perception that there is something missing. They see obstacles as temporary opportunities for growth and compassion. They don't expect sunshine everyday, and you might even find them dancing in the rain. They make the most of what ever is given them, and integrate it into a state of thankfulness. I was able to meet Dr. Emoto and be a presenter at one of the conventions he was also presenting at, and my turn to speak came right after his. How wonderful it was to further build on the foundation he already showed scientifically existed and was

233

possible; and then the miracle healings be an immediate real example of that possibility *being a reality*. It was inspiring to all!

The Inspiration of Music, Art, and Movement

At one point during my NDE I was standing before the core of His swirling presence - such a brilliant snapshot of the center of heaven - I was awaiting an answer to a question I had asked. I listened as hard as I could listen, waiting for His words. Then, just on the outside of my understanding, I faintly heard voices singing the most beautiful melody I had ever heard in my life. I felt a "knowing" that these were the blessed voices of those joined in the Great Amen, the Angels. I knew it was praise for Father, but I couldn't make out what the words were saying…though I could hear all the voices were in perfect melody and harmony, an entire range of perfection flowing through and around me. It was an exhilarating and deeply spiritual experience; and even more exciting when it happened later in time and I could here the words clearly, and the distinct layers of perfection in song and pure voice. Music is "on" full-time in heaven!

When Dr. Emoto set bottles of water on a table between two speakers, and exposed it to different kinds of music, he received some interesting findings. Uplifting classical music (such as Beethoven's Pastoral Symphony and Mozart's 40th) showed beautiful, symmetrical and multi-faceted crystals; whereas heavy-metal music, which is full of angry and vulgar words, produced crystals that were fragmented and malformed at best.

There are so many wonderful healers, remote viewers and intuitives I have found that are also artists and musicians. Whether their art is painting, embroidery, stained-glass, sewing, crocheting, clay, wood-working or boat-building, the intent of passion and love has forged a good channel between their mind, heart and hands. Musicians come in many varieties too – the mystic who has developed a well-trained ear but doesn't actually play an instrument, the singer whose instrument is her beautiful voice, the traditional fiddle player who plays by ear, the pianist who has 20 years of music theory – all fulfill a deep need for resonance in their soul, and to constantly immerse themselves to feel balanced and whole. There are many ways to balance.

In the world of movement, the ice-skater spins and jumps, the dancer twirls and the runner exceeds her personal best. Movement in the "zone" is often a creative process of physical inspiration. Is it any wonder that the flowing and emotional beauty of ice-skating ranks it as one of the top Olympic sports by millions of global viewers? Music, art and movement touches our spirit for inspiration in a way that mere words cannot, thus making it a perfect medium for articulating what cannot be expressed! These expressions of creativity lifts the spirit of all onlookers and produces another positive "ripple-effect" for the vibration of the entire world, and a further balancing of the soul who created it.

Learning to Pay Attention

Look at the small child squatting down into a little ball to look at the fuzzy red-and-black caterpillar crawling upon the ground. At this age, they have no desire to destroy it, but are simply in a state of "awe" and wanting to understand on its level. Children naturally commune with Divine a vibration of joy, excitement, and gratitude for all the splendors surrounding them. A small walk of simply going down the driveway to the mailbox is an adventure full of delightful details: the feel of satiny flower petals, the way the sun reflects off the wet rocks, the clouds formed like horses in the sky, the smell of the sage crushed by little fingers. There is so much we stop seeing when we grow up!

"...I tell you the truth, unless you change and become like little children, you will never enter the kingdom of heaven. Therefore whoever humbles himself like this child is the greatest in the kingdom of heaven." - Jesus (Mt. 18:3,4)

One of the best things that ever happened to me was having my own children; it allowed me to see again through the eyes of a child. It was such a gift, that even now, when my children are grown and not seeing the details anymore, their mother still is. I refuse to miss out on the adventure of texture, color, light and shade, sounds and smells, of the nature all around us. Even in the most crowded city, I have been able to find life blossoming through cracks in the cement, butterflies tasting the nectar of wild vines winding through trash heaps, and hummingbirds marking their successful passage with their notable whirl of wings, and I have noticed and loved them all.

When we make the time to see, *to really see,* we become co-creators with the Quantum Observer, and we help the world around us conform to Love's intentions. Do you want to live your entire life in someone else's perceptions and thoughtforms, or one of your own creation? *Become* the innocence of the mind of a child, look at the details, and see life finger-paint all of God's wonderful colors around and in your soul.

"...Mystics have long claimed to have a direct sense of contact with others, and if experiential knowledge of unity with all humans in all times. What are we to make of these claims? Are they conceivably valid? Although we have exquisite sensing abilities, our nervous systems are ingeniously clever at screening out stimuli - for instance, we are seldom aware of our clothes touching our skin. When we elect to do so, however, we can call into consciousness certain perceptions that are normally unconscious. For example, at any given moment we haven't the slightest idea what the bottom of our right foot feels like, yet on concentrating we begin to receive signals to tell us something about that area of our body. It is a matter of paying attention. Most of us learn to extinguish attention to external events. Aldous Huxley's "reducing valve" theory of consciousness still seems accurate: our consciousness, like an adjustable valve, set to allow only a very small fraction of stimuli reaching us to register in our mind. Yet our actual powers of sense perception are astonishing..." - Space, Time & Medicine by Larry Dossey, M.D.

This fraction of stimuli is one reason why the quiet of meditation and the connection of prayer helps us so much. When we quiet our mind, and focus on only a few things or even one, we can receive much more information without the white noise of everything else overlapping it. And, when we are able to quiet our mind to the place where focus is on the empty blackboard, and not on anything we ourselves have written upon it, that's when we will hear the voice of God, and His finger will write the message.

Solitude and Silence Promotes Insight

236

"I had no idea where I was going,
but, when I saw myself there,
great things did I understand...
of peace and of godliness was the perfect knowledge,
in profound solitude understood straight along;
it was something so secret,
that I was left stammering,
all knowledge transcending."

Excerpt from poem "I Entered Knowing Not Where"
by St. John of the Cross

Often, our sense of self and identity depends upon interaction both with the physical world and with other people. Removing ourselves voluntarily from the habits of how we *usually* interact with our environment helps us go into greater depth and awareness. We often get entrenched with our habits, for good or for bad. Looking at it from a third person sense gives us a new look at ourselves, and where we could make changes.

Silence is recognized by all cultures as a place where we can connect to mystery, where we can hear the whispers of the Great Eternal Soul. A good way of exploring this is to get away from present surroundings and see what emerges. Go camping, be out in nature; take some real time, and not just an hour or two. This should be a balanced period of time – only you will know if four days or 40 is what you need. But, as in many other things, it is not about quantity, but the quality of the time spent. Peace and receptivity are some wonderful shifts that promote balance and equilibrium. It is not about human "doing," but about human "being." When you have "come down from the mountain," you will have found new strength in your own voice emerged from the sound of silence. God speaks in whispers.

"That solitude promotes insight as well as change has been recognized by great religious leaders, who have usually retreated from the world before returning to it to share what has been revealed to them. Although accounts vary, the enlightenment which finally came to the Buddha whilst he was meditating beneath the tree on the banks of the Nairanjana river is said to

237

have been the culmination of long reflection upon the human condition. Jesus, according to both St. Matthew in St. Luke, spent forty days in the wilderness undergoing temptation by the devil before returning to proclaim the message of repentance and salvation. Mahomet, during the month of Ramadan, each year withdrew himself from the world to the cave Hera. St. Catherine of Siena spent three years in seclusion in her little room in the Via Benincasa during which she underwent a series of mystical experiences before entering upon an active life of teaching and preaching." – Solitude: A Return to Self by Anthony Storr

This sense of peace and friendship with silence brings us into a new reconciliation with ourselves and everything around us. It helps us know we belong to a greater whole, even when we return to our common life. Some religious mystics have a called this time of solitude *"waiting upon God."* This integration process has little to do with other people, because we desire a separate validity, an empirical experience. Hence, our most significant moments in which we attain new insight, and the moments of the most clarity, usually occur when we are in solitude and quiet, when we are truly *alone with the Alone.*

Awakening Begins with an In-The-Body Experience

In this shifting of the field of consciousness from lower to higher levels, your center of interest also changes. In this process of transcendence, you will come to a point where you realize that many of your habits are very limiting. Whereas your previous universe was organized around you, now you shift into the larger world-consciousness. In this expansion, the first place to go is *inside.* The first birth of the individual is into the deeper self, and this is where one finds a new breath that invigorates this new body; and the air is sweet!

This is when we see the Sunday *"Yard Sale"* signs go up, as simplicity is recognized as a greater need than the constant upkeep of things rarely used. This doesn't mean that living more spiritually equals a strictly austere or ascetic life of poverty or lack. In fact, abuses of this kind have sometimes given mysticism a name consistent with self-mutilation, deprivation and starvation. This is not the balance and wholeness true mysticism stands for.

238

But a desire for the simpler life means your focus has changed, and if you gathered material possessions as a sense of identity and value, you won't need them for that purpose anymore. In fact, once you have come to this place of realization, this is (comically) when the *abundance really starts to flow!* This abundance will not only include finances and material items, but also travel, vacation experiences, relationships and other intangible things too.

People who are in balance spiritually have certain qualities that shine forth in their personalities like luminous beacons in a foggy night. These people love without judging others, and understand that the Divine Spark is within every person, and they see each person as a child of God. They take responsibility for all they do and are very careful that their words and actions do not cause harm to others or to the earth. If they are not in some kind of career that involves service toward humanity, they often fill their off-hours in some way to help others and the earth. Whether it is helping to resolve problems in their neighborhood, environment or schools, or on the phone encouraging and supporting their many friends. They have a desire to help others and receive much satisfaction from it. They know who they are on the inside. They know how to give, and how to receive. *They know love!*

Spiritually balanced persons seem to be able to roll with the punches and come out on the other side unscathed. They come from a place of profound faith, and reliance on One greater than themselves. They will never be found guilty of gossiping, backbiting, cheating, blaming, faultfinding, or making any person feel inferior. They truly listen to others, are encouraging, tactful, humorous, humble, personable, compassionate and always willing to offer a listening ear or share a word of wisdom. They see their lives as being blessed and guided, have a sense of deep peacefulness. They look for Divine Coincidences every day of their lives. Truly enjoying life, they see every day as an adventure, and desire to consistently show unconditional love to every person they meet, as if they were meeting God himself. They accept each with tolerance and respect. They understand we walk alongside each other on our mutual journey of obtaining our true potential, of expanding into Love.

It doesn't matter if their physical body is whole or not - their spirit is, and others see it also and bask in the glow. What a wondrous life is theirs; and it's potentially attainable for every human on the planet, because it is part of every spirit's Free Will choice.

Coming Down from the Mountain and Out of the Cave – Service to Mankind

"These souls have a marked detachment from everything and a desire to be always either alone or busy with something that is to some soul's advantage." – Interior Castle by Teresa of Avila (16th century)

As we have seen, often the awakened soul yearns for the stillness, the place where tranquility and peace can take root and grow unimpeded. In previous times, and still in some parts of the world, there are people who go into isolation, into caves, and into monasteries and have little or no contact with the outside world. Some also take a vow of silence, or make a vow of another kind, often one that stretches the human capacity to the limit. Some stay in these places for all their lives. This is not the same as a wilderness vacation! However, many realize that to continue this kind of seclusion for extended periods of time *does little to truly advance their purpose towards receiving and expressing love.* You need *people* to do that, *interaction* with people.

We all have the same purpose. Jesus was questioned about 'what was the greatest commandment,' and he said, *"Love the Lord your God with all your heart and with all your soul and with all your mind and with all your strength...and Love your neighbor as yourself."* (Mk. 12:30,31) We just all have different ways, gifts and abilities to express this love. *Whatever brings you the most joy is your purpose!* Pursue the joy, and you will fulfill polishing the facets of love and connection you were made to be with yourself, others, and Him. Activate the joy in your life! Ask what makes you happy, and lift it up in *specific prayer* and Holy intention. Now see it manifest in front of you, recognizing two things as it appears: (1). God not only exists but cares about you and wants to interact with you because He loves you; (2). You can act on it and pursue it without fear since it is exactly what you prayed for, and let any doors close behind you as well, without fear.

To *love your neighbor as yourself* you have to know your neighbor, you have

240

to live actively in your life, and in the neighborhood. Only in this way will you truly feel a sense of purpose, as you interact as a positive change in your vicinity, and then going one step further, seeing the entire world as your next-door neighbor, a world community.

Indeed, activating the joy is a by-product of your love for your neighbor. And this applies to healing as well. Without true fellow-feeling and empathy, no healing would take place, either by hands-on or distant healing, since it is activated by passion and compassion.

"Healing grows out of the unconscious when a person is in rapport with the healing source. It is the ego, a function of the conscious mind, which blocks the experience of this rapport. The healer must unseat the ego without crushing it in order to open the doors to healing energy. Only then can rapport be established. Achieving rapport is accomplished by an act of surrender on the part of the healer; when the healer pushes aside the ego to make room for the I AM." – The Art of Spiritual Healing by Keith Sherwood

Jesus was an example of balance - he went into seclusion and quietness first - a 40 day trek into the desert wilderness while fasting and contemplating God, His purpose and His future. Then He came back, and began a ministry that was to forever change the world. He did not keep himself apart, but interacted with people at their level of comprehension, and went to their places of work and rest. He sat where people sat. *He met people at the point of their need.* He didn't preach a lot of sermons in the temple, but mostly in the streets, in the market place and in homes. He was driven by compassion and love and the conviction that He could make a difference, that He had an important purpose to his life, and that people needed to hear the message that He had to say. Jesus, among many other things, was also the truest of mystics, and worked hard in His world neighborhood. He still does.

Discover the Freedom of Sacred Attention

A courageous attitude is needed to fully navigate the mystical path. Often we will need to find the courage of a warrior in our battle to speak our truth no matter if it's accepted or not. It takes nerve to speak of things beyond the "normal" range of conversation, about the things that really matter. But this is when the greatest work is accomplished; this is how we *share enlightenment*. We have to be awake and paying attention to the flowing process, and the sacred presence of the full opportunity of the exact moment we are in.

"The present is the point where time touches eternity." – Father Kallistos Ware

What ever you are doing, be there to do it. Like the popular book by Eckhart Tolle says, there really is a lot to be said for *The Power of Now*. Discover the freedom of sacred attention; fully realize every flower bud, every bird song, every breeze on your skin and ray of sun on your face. Feel the depth and vibrations of the emotions that wave through you during the day, and put a name to each one. This way you will later recognize the tightness in your chest and the contraction in your stomach as fear, and be able to release and replace it. You will recognize the blush in your cheeks and warmth in your heart as love, and be able to express it, etc. Each emotion that you feel will be already known to you, and your ability to recognize which one as it comes, will do a lot with how to handle it. When you actually pay attention to your body/mind response to these emotions, familiarity and deeper perception replaces fear of the unknown.

As a mystic, you have experienced all emotions many times. You are in control with your choice of reaction to them. When you feel the heat of anger rising, you understand that you have control over this emotion. You can choose to dissipate it or follow it through to its negative cause-and-effect. But once you understand your emotions, you understand that you are the one in charge, and can rule them, and not the other way around. Understanding and being *in the moment* gives you this control.

The Art of Illumination, Seeing with New Eyes of Enlightenment

Playing with and appreciating children and animals, walking along the beach, camping in the mountains, listening to wonderful music, making love and making wine – all these things can bring the sacred life into a more wondrous fulfillment. And, it can be expanded the *how* you do it. The Uncreated Light manifests itself through the things that are created.

"I only went out for a walk and finally decided to stay until sundown, for going out I discovered was actually going in." – John Muir

Look at the redwood tree and embrace it with all your senses. You *see* what it looks like, now what does it *sound* like? The breezes filter a rustle of ten thousand branches, not like any other sound on earth! What does the redwood *feel* like? Manually touch its thick fibrous bark, notice the texture against your hand, and bury your nose into its sculpted crevices. What does it *smell* like? Notice the humus and ferns of a thousand years swirled at its feet, how it helps to check erosion and regulate climate. This is a true living being; breathing out huge clouds of oxygen, drinking hundreds of gallons of water, bridging earth and sky, birds and earthworms, plants and insects.

Notice that this is much more than just a tree; feel the deep rest and peace of this living being, and bring it into yourself. See your feet diving down into the fertile soil like rootlets thrusting forward for moisture and nutrients, envision your arms as uppermost branches embracing the sun and rain, bird and squirrel. Be aware of the radiance and perfection of this single universe right here in front of you. The tree has invited you into its electromagnetic field, and its energy tracing has now dusted you, as yours has also dusted the tree. You have communed together, two living beings alone together in the active stillness…

A question to ask yourself, - do you impact your neighborhood as positively as this redwood does? Do you convert the pollution around you (profanity, lewd behavior, depression, anger) into a whole new item, actually exchanging it for something useful (helpful encouragement, manners, joy, love)? Though you cannot control the Free Will of others, you can transcend the effects of shadow and transform it into light. In the same way, you can activate change in all aspects of the vibrational pattern of matter, which science has shown is only slowed down energy. With this information and attention to detail, and the ability to surrender in the Cosmic embrace of the high energy of Divine Love, all things are possible to experience, and to change. This is the place where spoons bend, healing miracles occur, abundance manifests, and the river

243

of infinite knowledge becomes accessible. You now have a glimmer of the mind of God, and your true mind as well.

"By the law of congruency you can control your environment and you can transcend the reaches of cosmos. By mentally stimulating the atomic pattern and then becoming that pattern by the adjustment of your consciousness, you can walk through a garden wall, enter into the heart of a flower of journey to the depths of the sea. You can become all things, know all things...I AM thy God. Thou art in me, and I AM in thee. We are one through that point of contact...when you understand, you will experience a million miracles and in so doing bless the entire sphere of your consciousness." – The Masters and the Spiritual Path by Elizabeth and Mark Prophet

The majestic eagle high upon the desert escarpment believes in grace. No fear in believing what can't be seen, she jumps off the cliff onto the invisible safety net of the embrace of the air. She does not ponder black or white questions about flight, there are no grey in-between answers that may or may not be true. Everything just IS. And everything IS as it should be. Where eagles soar, you can too. For those who will let it happen and not flinch or draw back, any barriers of perceived fear dissolves and you can feel what the bird feels, you can ask to be "one" with that consciousness.

You can just as easily release and go out of body into the space of your living room as you can in the woodlands above your town, or in your city park. And instead of feeling and tasting the plasterboard and insulation of the ceiling as you move through it, why not choose to experience a tree, an animal, a bird? You can you know! The spark of consciousness of who you are is part of the same Flame that created all this to begin with. The same way that we can live in and experience such things, is the same way we can live in and experience Divine Love.

"No one has ever seen God, but if we love one another, God lives in us and his love is made complete in us. We know that we live in him and he in us, because he has given us of his Spirit...God is love. Whoever lives in love lives in God, and God in him." (1 John 4:12 -13, 16)

244

Once you have made the transition in opening to the True Energy, you will learn that self-discovery never ends. With the acknowledgement of self connection in this fabric of life, self-discovery becomes discovery of all things. It never ends! And it never gets boring! Everything is truly possible when you recognize you are a co-creator in the holographic mind of God.

Healing the World through Mindful Intent

"I look at God as the Grandest of Engineers, the power behind the movement of stars in the one extreme, to warm winds on a summer night in the other. It is our spiritual relationship with God that brings purpose to our interface with reality." – The Ultimate Time Machine by Joesph McMoneagle

"Our ability to experience personal communication beyond the physical is profoundly self-empowering. As we grow in this ability, we are better able to expand the ways we perceive and communicate with the unseen worlds around us. Eventually we will reach a point where we become a spiritual explorer who is fully aware of and consciously interacting with the other dimensions of reality. I believe the increasing number of people around the world who are beginning to explore and cultivate this ability represents a major leap in the development and evolution of human consciousness." –The Secret of the Soul by William Buhlman

We live at a time of great opportunity. Mankind is at the cutting edge of bridging the gap between both worlds: the seen and the unseen, ancient and modern, conventional and integrative medicine, and science and spirituality. Advances in science coupled with increased communication have created new paradigms of thinking and moving in our ever-dependent world. As such, what one nation does is felt strongly by all others. And what each individual does in those nations develops the structure and countenance that is reflected in that nation. More than ever before, the choice of each individual has a noticed culminate effect to manifest change in the world, for good or for bad. And though we have TV, radio and print to magnify the *word* of these changes, the invisible vibration of our neighbors have been surrounding us everyday, and we continue to be affected by the *feel* of it.

245

As we have seen, we can change the world by changing our intentions and mind-set. What are the possible implications of that? We can heal and see miracles in mind and body, in-person or by distance. We can remote view, alone and together as groups, to locate a missing child. We can intuit previously undiagnosable medical conditions, and help target conventional medicine to the problem. We can literally do anything; nothing is beyond our grasp, when we allow the oneness of our positive flow to intermingle with the Ultimate Positive Force.

"Each particle of mass in our bodies represents one closure of the entire universe – yielding a holographic reality – and deeper communication with ourselves is identical to communication with the universe, including any part of it, at any distance. Furthermore, in hyperspace the future and the past are all present. Since a particle does indeed exhibit a four-dimensional component for 1/137 of the time, each particle does connect to the future and to the past. With selective tuning and kindling any part of this holographic reality is accessible. However, because of the smallness of a single selective signal in the midst of the totality, the channel is quite noisy.- The Ecstasy is Here Now! by Bearden, 1988.

There is a floating existence of being in the freedom and fulfillment which flows from unity in the Spirit. It is spontaneous full enjoyment of life, and is beyond words. A person can live in a physical body and still experience the complete unity and knowledge of the Spirit. It is actually an experiencing of the contents of heaven in love.

As your mystical unfolding, blossoming and foundation building continues, many wonderful things beyond ordinary comprehension are going to follow. Perhaps healing miracles will occur spontaneously in your presence, or you may attract highly realized humans to bilocate to you for a chat, or you to them. Perhaps you will have precognition of a destructive event and be able to lessen its duration or intensity through intention and specific prayer. Be passionate about it, and it will positively happen.

"Praise be to the name of God for ever and ever…He gives wisdom to the wise and knowledge to the discerning. He reveals deep and hidden things; he

246

knows what lies in darkness, and light dwells with him" (Da. 2:20-22)

"...There is a God in Heaven Who Reveals Mysteries." (Da. 2:28)

I have endeavored to encourage you along your journey. Now you will continue along the path, not on your own, but with other people, information and adventures brought in to help you continue. I hope my sharing with you has allowed you to further push all fear and stagnation aside, and help you recognize the Love that you are and that you move and live in and toward. It has been an honor for me to accompany you for this segment of your ride. And please recognize that this book has been offered to you as a road map, and a love letter...be blessed!

A Fellow Traveler,
Tiffany Snow

Stargate of the Mind

The Stargate of the mind
Reaches past the barrier of frontiers.
In an iridescent chariot of fire,
The lucid pioneer
Races by in his astral body.

The paradigm shift
Of bumping my head on the ceiling
Not a few times
A view mirrored anciently by saints
And yogis alike,
Is the resonance beyond gravity,
Beyond casual words.

Laws change in the Stargate,
New realities are expanded
As is the human intent.
Stretched like a new wineskin,
It ferments the drink
And intoxicates our senses,
And we yearn for more visions.

Allow yourself
The insane silliness to see beyond,
And to discover that deep space is never empty,
Love can take us through any barrier,
And ceilings only exist in a mind
That is fearful of stars.

Other Books by Tiffany Snow

THE POWER OF DIVINE: A HEALER'S GUIDE
-Tapping into the Miracle

ISBN:0-9729623-3-6 SPIRITJOURNEYBOOKS.COM

COME INTO THE WORLD OF MIRACLES!

WINNER OF 3 AWARDS! San Diego Book Awards - USA BOOKNEWS AWARDS - Reader's Preference Editor's Choice Awards

"Standing at center stage at the intersection of science, religion and healing you will find Tiffany Snow's newest book "The Power of Divine." *This is one of the most interesting books on the market today* when it comes to understanding the importance of prayer in the healing process. Focusing on divine healing where the healer prayerfully calls on direct intervention by God, it is a trip into the world of miracles and how prayer changes lives." **MIDWEST BOOK REVIEW; Dr. Harold D. McFarland, PhD editor** *Readers Preference Reviews*

"Tiffany Snow gets to the point. Do you want to be a healer of yourself and others? Here is a road map to help you find your way, as I had to find mine. The healer's guide she outlines is what I describe as "questions I have never thought of." Socrates would have applauded her."- **Rev. Francis J. Marcolongo, S.T.L., S.S.L., Ph.D.**

"Tiffany Snow is both a gift, and a giver of gifts. Her book, "THE POWER OF DIVINE: A HEALER'S GUIDE – TAPPING INTO THE MIRACLE," is an awesome guide to healing from a masterful healer/author. Tiffany has created a comprehensive manual on tapping into the Source within, and finding the miracles that divine power can bring. Whether you are a Christian or not, whether you believe in God or a Force of Life, this is a powerful and inspiring book that documents the amazing healing energies available to all of us. Her book is filled with powerful and profound stories of healing, scientific and medical research, and plenty of information on how to facilitate true healing for yourself and others. This is a wonderful book and should be on the shelf of any spiritual seeker who truly wants to improve their own life, as well as the world as a whole. Kudos to Tiffany Snow for providing us with all the tools we could possibly need to become healers and positive forces for good in the world." - **Rev. Marie Jones, Author of LOOKING FOR GOD IN ALL THE WRONG PLACES**

"Dr. Snow has simply done a marvelous job! "The Power of Divine" is packed full of inspiration, with many heartwarming and poignant stories of how God works in human lives. Each section of a chapter can be used as an excellent guide for group reflection and discussion to help people understand more clearly how God could be working in their own lives. Thank you, Tiffany for your lovely book and the huge endeavor it represents!" – **James P. O'Conner, Director of CSCS/ Center for Spirituality and Community Stewardship**

"Medical Spirituality at it's best. Put "THE POWER OF DIVINE: A HEALER'S GUIDE" on your summer reading list. I had heard many things about this book from my co-workers, so was anxious to read it for myself. I was pleasantly surprised that the hype stood the test! I have never found a nonfiction book so calming to read, where the author makes you feel that you are in the kitchen sharing a cup of tea & cookies - while easily getting down to the roots of illness, emotional problems, and what to do about it. There is humor here, balanced with spirituality that goes beyond religion. Prayer and conventional medicine combined together could really be the shape of the future in health care, and according to Dr. Snow, that future is starting to be realized now, and we can have a "hand" in it. Excellent Q & A chapter too. A Must Read." - **Monica Farrington, R.N.**

"This is an excellent discussion of spiritual healing, for both healers and healees. Tiffany Snow started her working career writing songs and producing records in Nashville, Tennessee. Her now considerable healing gifts were awakened after being struck by lightning and having a near-death experience. She has become a minister and regularly offers healing in church as well as in individual sessions. People often lose consciousness when they receive healing, entering ecstatic states which are classically described as being 'slain in the spirit.'

What I like about Snow's book is her practical, down to earth attitude, and her openness to learning herself from her work. While herself practicing firmly within a Christian tradition, Snow is respectful of other healing traditions. Snow has a gift for sharing profound observations in light-hearted manners. She comments on the complexity of human relationships and the healings that may extend beyond the person presenting with symptoms or illnesses. This book is a good read, in addition to its informative content. Warmly recommended for anyone interested in healing."
- Daniel J. Benor, M.D., Author of SPIRITUAL HEALING – Scientific Validation of A Healing Revolution

QUICK ORDER FORM

THE POWER OF DIVINE: A HEALER'S GUIDE
-Tapping into the Miracle

ISBN:0-9729623-3-6 SPIRITJOURNEYBOOKS.COM

For orders via mail, please send this form along with check or money order
Written to: Spirit Journey Books

Spirit Journey Books
P.O. Box 61
San Marcos, CA 92079
1-800-535-5474

For expedited orders, please order via our secure credit card link at our websites:

www.SpiritJourneyBooks.com
www.TiffanySnow.com

Name:_____

Address:_____

City:_____State:_____Zip:_____

Email or phone number:_____

Amount for each Book is: $18.95   Book $18.95
                                                   (Quantity) x (   )
CA. Sales Tax: (7.75% If applicable)   +CA. Tax   (   )
                                                   +Shipping   (   )

                                                   TOTAL=_____

Shipping: Please add $3.00 for first book, and $1.00 each additional book.
Tax: Please add 7.75% for books shipped to California addresses.

253

Other Books by Tiffany Snow

PSYCHIC GIFTS IN THE CHRISTIAN LIFE - Tools to Connect

ISBN:0-9729623-0-1 SPIRITJOURNEYBOOKS.COM

ACTIVATE SPIRITUAL GIFTS IN YOUR DAILY LIFE!

"Tiffany Snow's *PSYCHIC GIFTS IN THE CHRISTIAN LIFE - TOOLS TO CONNECT* is the book you've been waiting for. It is a "self-help" manual that will show you how to manifest and use your Supernatural Gifts. Step-by-step learn how to tap into the Divine Connection and your own natural-born intuitive abilities.Each reading of this amazing book will lead you to a new level of understanding, ability and insight for enhancing your self and God awareness and for the betterment of the world."
- Ivy Helstein, Psychotherapist and Author of *INFINITE ABILITIES: Living Your Life On Purpose*

FINALLY! A book that speaks frankly about God's Supernatural Gifts as a NATURAL AND NORMAL PART OF SPIRITUAL LIFE!

"Thank you, Tiffany, for being in the world and for helping it to be a better place for all of us to be. God bless...I am proud of the work you are so diligently doing in service to enlightenment. Keep it up, Girlfriend. The world is a much better place due to the loving efforts of shining souls such as yourself." - **Dannion Brinkley, International Best-Selling Author of *Saved By the Light, At Peace in the Light*, and Founder of Compassion in Action**

"Through Tiffany's sharing of her amazing journey, she is a pioneer in bridging religion with spirituality, reminding us all that life is about our own experience and expression of the powerful love of God in our everyday life. It is a must read for all people on all paths of life."- **Joan Grinzi, RN, President of Holistic Health Resources/*Alternative Paths to Healing***

"Tiffany Snow has written a remarkably lucid presentation of how to make the Spirit and spiritual gifts each of us possesses become activated in our daily lives. Besides being a "How-To-Book" it is more importantly an invitation, a clarion call to "why not you?" **Rev. Francis J. Marcolongo, S.T.L., S.S.L., Ph.D., MFT**

"Tiffany Snow is as gifted a writer as she is a healer. Her book, "Psychic Gifts in the Christian Life: Tools to Connect," is filled with wisdom, insight and a pure spiritual joy that is infectious. She is truly an inspiration; a bright light in a world so often filled with darkness."- **Rev. Marie D. Jones, Author** *of Looking For God In All The Wrong Places*

From the Author: Tiffany says: "From the very beginning, God has demonstrated that his Spirit is Supernatural, and has given us gifts to keep in contact with him. So many of us have special abilities that are shut down as children, from well-meaning friends or misinformed religions. But God has always used Supernatural ways to connect with his kids, and still does today. Become the potential you already are! In my book, GOD IS OUT OF THE BOX! And, for those who are Christian, throughout the book you will find cited scriptural backing for understanding your gifts without fear. No one has to be struck by *lightning* to have this Connection – my hope is that this book will be *your* defining moment. We ALL have gifts!"

From a sumptuous buffet laid before you, you will be able to choose from many tools to learn how to use and develop the natural gifts we were all created with, and the Supernatural ones that we can tap into. Games will activate your God-Spots becoming more intuitive and sensitive. Some Topics: Channeling Holy Spirit; Finding Missing Children through Prayer Power, Helping the FBI, our God-Spots.

QUICK ORDER FORM

Psychic Gifts in the Christian Life – Tools to Connect

ISBN:0-9729623-0-1 SPIRITJOURNEYBOOKS.COM

For orders via mail, please send this form along with check or money order
Written to: Spirit Journey Books

Spirit Journey Books
P.O. Box 61
San Marcos, CA 92079
1-800-535-5474

For expedited orders, please order via credit card through our websites at:

www.SpiritJourneyBooks.com
www.TiffanySnow.com

Name:_____

Address:_____

City:_____State:_____Zip:_____

Email or phone number:_____

Amount for Book is: $24.95

CA. Sales Tax: (7.75% If applicable)

Book	$24.95
(Quantity) x	( )
+CA. Tax	( )
+Shipping	( )

TOTAL=_____

Shipping: Please add $3.00 for first book, and $1.00 each additional book.
Tax: Please add 7.75% for books shipped to California addresses.

Thank you God! Amen!

Printed in the United States
67812LVS00005B/151-153